The Nursing Home Decision

The Nursing Home Decision

Easing the Transition for Everyone

Lawrence M. Martin, M.D.

Consultant, Division of Adult Psychiatry,
Mayo Clinic and Mayo Foundation; Assistant
Professor of Psychiatry, Mayo Medical School;
Rochester, Minnesota

John Wiley & Sons, Inc.
New York • Chichester • Weinheim • Brisbane • Singapore • Toronto

This publication is designed to provide accurate and authoritative information in regard to the subject matter covered. It is sold with the understanding that the publisher is not engaged in rendering professional services. If professional advice or other expert assistance is required, the services of a competent professional person should be sought.

ISBN: 0-471-34804-X

Printed in the United States of America

10   9   8   7   6   5   4   3   2   1

To Lois

For the inspiration and perspiration
May I have the privilege of growing older with you

Contents

Acknowledgments

My wife, who provided not only the original idea but the ongoing support and encouragement to complete this project.

The residents, past and present, of the skilled nursing facilities at Rochester Samaritan Bethany Home on Eighth; Charterhouse, Inc (retirement community); Woodside/Aspen Care and Rehabilitation Center; and the Sisters of St. Francis at Assisi Heights, who have been and continue to be my best teachers.

My parents, who, at age 83, continue to reassure me about the future with their own vitality, continued growth, and active planning for their future.

My daughters, who I hope not to burden with decisions that I could have made and who remind me to plan for my own future rather than theirs.

Roberta J. Schwartz, LeAnn M. Stee, Marlené M. Boyd, Dorothy L. Tienter, and Dr. Carol L. Kornblith of the Section of Publications, Mayo Clinic and Mayo Foundation, who have helped me through the jungles of editing and preparing this book for publication.

The Nursing Home Decision

Introduction

The period surrounding a move to a nursing home is a difficult time. It is usually a decision that is forced on the person, family, and friends by medical and situational problems that can no longer be managed in any other way. It may make real those things that we would like to deny about people we love—that they are older, sicker, and not the same as we would like or need them to be.

It is hard to prepare ourselves for such an experience. We may be surprised at the strong and mixed reactions we feel during the decision-making, entry, and settling-in processes. Much attention has been focused on the way new nursing home residents adapt to this change. Less has been paid to the stresses experienced by close family and friends. No book can change the things families must go through. However, it is often said that "knowledge is power." This simply means that the more we understand about what is happening, the less frightened and powerless we will feel.

This book is designed to help the family and friends of the prospective or new nursing home resident. It also will help nursing home staff who are asked to make the new resident and the family feel welcomed, safe, and, eventually, at home.

The first part of the book describes some of the common tasks and problems as seen from different viewpoints: the new resident, the family and friends, and the staff of the nursing home. The second part looks at opportunities for managing these tasks. Although most of us will read from our own perspective, reading others' viewpoints will help us to understand and share the burdens of this time.

This book is not intended to be a textbook. It does not pretend to offer specific solutions to the difficult management problems often found. Nothing can substitute for a caring team involving physicians, nurses, social workers, occupational and physical therapists, psychologists, clergy, nurses' aides, family, and friends. All play important roles in the care of the resident and each other.

Chapter 1

Why a Nursing Home?

Nursing homes (sometimes called "rest homes," "convalescent centers," or "care centers") are not new. They are in some ways an outgrowth of the old "county home." This was usually a small institution within the community that housed people with nowhere else to go: the chronically mentally ill, the mentally retarded, the alcoholic, the indigent, and the elderly without family. The care was mostly custodial—shelter and food. These homes were funded by the community and seen as a community resource and responsibility.

Current nursing homes bear little resemblance to these early institutions. At times looking more like acute care hospitals, today's nursing homes are expected to care for residents with complex medical and behavioral problems. Care is provided by a team that includes nurses (registered and practical), nurses' aides, nurse practitioners, physicians, social workers, therapists (physical, occupational, speech, and recreational), housekeepers, administrators, clergy, volunteers, and family members. Each plays an important and different role.

Why has there been such a growth in the number of

nursing homes and such dramatic changes in the level of care given in nursing homes? There are several reasons that will become even more important in the years ahead.

First, we are getting older. The fastest growing segment of the population is people older than age 85. Illnesses that used to kill people in their early or middle years are now prevented (for example, vaccination for polio) or better treated (for example, antibiotic drugs for pneumonia and insulin for diabetes). We are now better able to control conditions that contribute to potentially fatal illnesses. The discovery and medical management of high blood pressure and high blood cholesterol level decrease the likelihood of stroke and heart attack. We are starting to take better care of ourselves (for example, by stopping smoking, eating healthier diets, and exercising). We are paying more attention to safety at work, in our cars, and at home. These changes are all positive, but they mean that more of us will be old.

Second, more people survive with illnesses and conditions that require nursing home care. People may survive an illness, such as a stroke or a heart attack because of better medical care, but be disabled and require ongoing nursing home care. People also are more likely to suffer from the disabilities of the elderly, such as vision and hearing loss, osteoporosis, and Alzheimer's disease.

Tracy Kidder described this mixed blessing in the book *Old Friends*. Earl had a massive heart attack.

> By feeding an array of drugs into his bloodstream, the doctors brought Earl to a stable condition, and eventually they sent him home. A few weeks later, though, he was rushed to the hospital. This pattern held through the summer, fall, and early winter. Earl would spend a week or two . . . on the verge of death—from heart arrhythmias, from cardiac

arrest, from congestive heart failure, from intramural thrombus ... and, mainly because his heart had become an inadequate pump, from fulminant pneumonia and kidney failure. Again and again the cardiac unit staff brought him back, with oxygen therapy, with a pacemaker, with drugs that lessen, in various ways, the work that the heart has to do. Again and again Earl rallied, and his doctors sent him home with a virtual pharmacopoeia—digoxin, Capoten, Lasix, Quinaglute, Zaroxolyn, Coumadin, potassium chloride, sublingual nitroglycerin ...

Only a decade or so before, Earl would probably have died shortly after his heart attack. The steady advance of cardiac pharmacology deserved much of the credit, perhaps also the blame, for his having survived these last six months.

Third, there are fewer caregivers and they are not as available. According to Schlepp (see Readings on page 19), 13 percent of the population will be older than age 65 by the year 2000, with the number increasing to 20 percent by the year 2050. Our society is no longer a rural one. The norm for previous generations—a larger family with children staying on the farm or living close by after growing up—was a built-in support for an elderly parent in failing physical or mental health. Women were often at home. Several adult children shared the burden in a familiar environment. The extended family served to support those providing care as well as the person in need.

Life is very different than this for most of us. As children grow up, they tend to move away. It is increasingly common for an older person to have no responsible relative living close by. This means that the older person may face a choice of staying alone in familiar surroundings or moving to a new, unfamiliar place to be near family. Family members are not as present in the home. Schlepp noted, "People who care for aging parents usually are female between the ages of 40 and 60. Two thirds of the caregivers are married, and more than one half are employed either full time (42%) or part time (13%)."

Fourth, people are being dismissed from the hospital sooner. Increasing costs of health care and regulations from government and private insurance companies mean that everyone, including the elderly, tends to be dismissed from hospitals sooner. This particularly affects older people, who tend to heal more slowly, are more likely to have multiple medical problems, have complications from medicines and other treatment, and have fewer and less vigorous caregivers at home. German and colleagues reported that nearly two-thirds of all new nursing home residents are admitted directly from the hospital. Some convalesce and some die, but both German (et al.) and Simms (et al.) found that between one-half and two-thirds are still living in the nursing home after one year.

Although estimates suggest that only 5 percent of people older than age 65 are in nursing homes at any specific moment, the number of elderly who will at some point require this level of care is much higher, with estimates reported by German (et al.) as ranging from 20 percent to 50 percent. I recently surveyed obituaries listing place of death and found that almost 50 percent of individuals died in nursing homes (Martin LM, unpublished data). This same survey noted that each person dying in a nursing home had an average of three to four first-degree relatives (spouse and children). The number of survivors would increase significantly if grandchildren and friends were included.

The implication of the above statistics and patterns is clear: the nursing home has become a necessary part of the lives of an increasing number of Americans.

Readings

German PS, Rovner BW, Burton LC, Brant LJ, Clark R: "The Role of Mental Morbidity in the Nursing Home Experience." *The Gerontologist* 32:152–158, 1992

Kidder T: *Old Friends.* New York, Houghton Mifflin Company, 1993, pp 108–109

Schlepp S: "Elder Care. Caregiving—Learning to Cope, Learning the Options." *AORN Journal* 50:228–236, 1989

Simms LM, Jones SJ, Yoder KK: "Adjustment of Older Persons in Nursing Homes." *Journal of Gerontological Nursing* 8:383–386, 1982

Chapter 2

The Image

The nursing home has a lingering image problem. It has been called a warehouse for the elderly. Some people imply that it is a place where uncaring or selfish children or spouses put relatives who are unwanted or in the way. There is a perception that only custodial care is provided and that this care is of poor quality. The staff of the nursing home is often pictured as poorly trained and uncaring, frequently neglecting and sometimes abusing the vulnerable residents. Many people associate nursing homes with old age, failing physical and mental strength, and death. Nursing homes have not been places to look toward with anticipation for potential residents or the people close to them. And, after all, aren't we all potential residents?

Several things contribute to this bad image. First, there are situations where some of the above problems do occur. As much as we would like to believe that everyone cares about those people who have been an important part of our lives, there are some who may not have that capacity. This may be difficult for us to understand, because we are taking the time to better understand and deal with this hard situation. Although there are some individuals who just are too self-absorbed to be involved in this process, there are usually other reasons for withdrawal or lack of involvement. These reasons will be described in more detail in Chapter 6.

Just as there are family members who aren't caring, there are individual staff members who are not well suited to work in long-term care. These individuals may have trouble with impulse control, they may want or need immediate results, or they may see the residents as worthless (see "ageism" in Chapter 3) and therefore see their own work as meaningless. They may deal with their sense of frustration or feelings of ineffectiveness, particularly with the behaviors of those residents with dementia, by blaming the residents. Most people are aware of stories of gross abuse or neglect by nursing home employees. In some ways, the less obvious incidents may be even more disquieting, in that they might be more likely to be ongoing and less likely to be reported. Rough handling during necessary care, demeaning comments, and, perhaps the most common, neglect of emotional needs do not spring from a single source. Limited personnel, little training in the specific disease processes as well as in basic human emotional needs and coping techniques, administrative or financial constraints, and lack of regular medical supervision all may contribute to problems in care.

Frequently those in the caring professions point the finger at those in other disciplines—at the physician who doesn't come often enough, at the nurse who administrates but doesn't see the residents day to day, or at the nurse's aide for the lack of professional training and rough treatment of residents. Sadly, one individual may harm the residents and the trust of the community in the entire institution.

Second, the poor image has some of its origins in memories of the old county home. The implications of poverty and having no one to care for us are not how we wish to be remembered. We all hope to be seen as respectable and successful. Ideally, most of this positive sense comes from inside ourselves. Yet, others' opinions of us remain important—a reason why we spend time and money to maintain our homes, cars, and clothing. The move to a nursing home may bring with it a loss of sense of respectability for the resident and the family. It is a great irony that the expense of being in a nursing home may create poverty.

Third, the move to the nursing home makes real many unspoken fears for all involved. Declining health or memory or the reality of oncoming death is something we tend to deny about a loved one or ourselves. The necessity of moving to a nursing home makes this denial more difficult. Because the obvious change is the living setting, we tend to blame it for our discomfort and anxiety. The unfair but impassioned demand, "Promise me you will never put me in a nursing home!" may well have its origins in these fears.

We make many of our decisions on the basis of our assumptions and expectations. If our belief is that the nursing home setting is bad, wrong, or evil, we may respond accordingly. If we are the prospective residents, we may refuse, withdraw, or become "bitter-enders," postponing the decision, preparations, and arrangements until someone else is forced to do these things for us.

The same may be true of family. We may wait until we are forced to make hasty decisions without much information or investigation. Although there are some medical situations that are truly unpredictable, many times an evolving situation or diagnosis may provide adequate warning that nursing home placement will likely be necessary. An obvious example is that of a person with Alzheimer's disease. The progression of the condition is well known. The steadily increasing requirements for physical care and supervision are the rule rather than the exception. Yet often the need to pursue nursing home placement seems abrupt, as if it were unforeseen. This procrastination limits the family's opportunity to investigate different options, visit different facilities, and speak with staff and family members of other residents.

Can we change our negative image of all nursing homes? This seems a lot to ask. However, the unknown makes fears worse. The more knowledge we have, the more realistic our concerns and the more appropriate our choices. Perhaps a reasonable goal is to see the nursing home for what it is: a necessary and appropriate care setting for many people with difficult health problems run by people like ourselves, who are fallible but caring and with good intentions, who have specialized medical knowledge.

A special note should be made of the term "resident" to describe the individual in the nursing home. Terminology can be important. Just as modern medicine has struggled because of positive and negative implications with the label "patient" to describe an individual who comes for care, the term "resident" also has both positive and negative implications. A resident is someone living at a given place, not passing through. This helps distinguish between a nursing home and an acute care hospital. However, it may devalue the serious illnesses or conditions that led the individual to require the setting of the nursing home in the first place. In this book the common term "resident" has been chosen, but not without concern about the need to acknowledge that most residents are suffering from illnesses that require ongoing supervision and treatment.

Chapter 3

No One Likes Getting Old

Do you remember when you couldn't wait to be older? Time between birthdays seemed endless. Each year meant greater knowledge, physical strength and coordination, privileges, and opportunities. Being older gave us more freedom—to play outside without supervision, to bathe ourselves, to not have a specific bedtime, to date, to drive, to live away from our parents' home, to get a job, to drink, to marry, and to have children. These freedoms all required age, and the older the better. What happened?

Getting older is not as simple as it sounds. It is certainly more than passively watching time go by on a clock or a calendar. Most of us acknowledge that seconds, days, months, and years are exactly the same duration as when we were children, yet our time sense is very different as adults. Time now seems to pass with lightning quickness. "Where have the years gone?" is an often-asked and seldom-answered question.

Our experience of getting older changes as well. No longer do we look forward to birthdays as evidence of getting older. Although the day itself may still be enjoyable because we are treated specially, the increasing years start to become an enemy.

We handle this change with differing levels of maturity. At one extreme is the person who experiences increasing age with feelings of satisfaction at things learned or better understood. This person has a sense of accomplishment in work and relationships and anticipates further self-understanding as a unique and changing individual. This person finds that these experiences compensate for losses in physical vigor and attractiveness. In the book *Songs of Experience*, Polly Francis, a fashion illustrator and photographer, wrote of her aging experience at age 92.

> In earlier times I didn't look beyond the move of the moment. Each move seemed almost fixed and final. But now all feeling of permanency has slipped away . . . . A new set of faculties seems to be coming into operation. I seem to be awakening to a larger world of wonderment—to catch little glimpses of the immensity and diversity of creation. More than at any other time in my life, I seem to be aware of the beauties of our spinning planet and the sky above. And now I have the time to enjoy them. I feel that old age sharpens our awareness.

At the other extreme is the individual whose denial of growing older is so profound that it manifests itself in embarrassing behavior. The middle-aged woman dressed in a miniskirt and dramatically groomed in a hairstyle or color appropriate to a teenager or the paunchy man in a mid-life crisis who leaves his wife and family for a motorcycle and a woman 20 years his junior may be demonstrating this denial.

Most of us are somewhere in between. Men attempt to play the sports of their youth and cannot get out of bed the next day. They secretly worry over thinning hair and their part drops toward the ear. They enjoy the successes of their children without living through them. Women fret over their stretch marks, the inability to attain the impossible slimness deemed attractive in our culture, and their daughters' choosing different values and not wanting them to be their best friend (but rather, their mother). They find things to value about themselves beyond physical attractiveness and the ability to sacrifice for others. Mostly, we do pretty well.

Chronological age is important and seems different for the different sexes. Age 30 seems more traumatic for women than men. In a culture that values women for physical attractiveness and idealizes slenderness, women older than age 30 may feel they cannot compete. Success for women is still all too often measured by their ability to attract men. Age can then quickly become a threat to security, lovableness, and a sense of control over one's future.

For men, age 40 may be a trial. Our culture tends to value men less for physical prowess (professional athletes excepted) and appearance than for material success. This can take the form of money or income, possessions, position or title, or fame. All of these imply increased power, dominance, and specialness. By age 40, men tend to evaluate themselves on the basis of these measures of success.

For both men and women transition birthdays are often celebrated with mock funeral services and over-the-hill parties featuring black balloons and gag gifts implying old age, such as laxatives, denture adhesives, and hair dye. Underneath this heavy-handed humor are the unspoken expectations of the inevitable downhill slide into old age and the death of youth, vigor, productivity, and attractiveness. Yet the odds are high that 40-year-olds have more than half of their life span yet to live.

Our society fears and seeks to avoid old age. Most of us

have redefined "old" or "elderly" several times, each time using an age that is older than our own.

There are examples everywhere. The author grew up in the generation whose battle cry was "Don't trust anyone over 30!"—as if no one would ever reach this dreaded age and become, by definition, untrustworthy.

A 77-year-old woman seen for evaluation of depression complained of a chronic sense of loneliness and isolation. When the interviewer naïvely inquired whether the individual had visited the local senior citizens' center, the patient replied, "I went there once, but there was nothing but old people . . . no one I could relate to."

The elderly are frequently the objects of derision, particularly when it comes to sexuality. The virile "young studs" ogling bikini-clad women in beer commercials are performing the identical behavior that earns older men the label "dirty old men." We often speak to the elderly as if they are children, choosing simple words in short sentences and speaking in a loud voice. The young woman who speaks up and stands by her convictions is seen as assertive. The older woman doing the same thing is often called crotchety. Perhaps no society reveres youth and reviles the elderly as much as ours does. There are stereotyped views of older people as unattractive, unproductive, weak, unintelligent, and asexual. The elderly are seen as worth less in our country.

A detailed examination of these stereotypes of the elderly (often called "ageism") is not our goal in this book. Ageism may have its origins in the youthfulness of our society. American culture is only a few hundred years old and is made up of individuals whose ancestors (African-Americans excepted, who didn't come by choice) placed greater importance on making a better life for themselves and their children than they did on tradition. This group may well have seen their elders as poor, ineffective, and downtrodden. The American dream is based on the presumption that we each make our own way and that we expect each succeeding generation to do even better. There is not much room in this setting to respect, listen to, or value elders. We may be too busy living up to the expectations of achievement taught to us by our elders.

Another potential cause for these commonly held attitudes toward the elderly may be found in the secular nature of our culture. All religions provide an explanation for our existence, a code of conduct for our life, and a way to understand our death. The promised Hereafter, whether the reincarnation and circular view of Hinduism or the Heaven of the Judeo-Christian religions, offers us the security of continuing on. A secular view offers one chance at life. Getting older represents getting closer to ceasing to exist. It makes sense that this would be frightening and something to be denied and avoided.

The dilemma of ageism is that, with the passage of time, we become what in our youth we denied, reviled, or ridiculed. Seldom are people forced to become a member of a group about which they have had prejudice (for example, gender, racial, ethnic, or religious prejudice). Our stereotypes remain safe in the differences that don't change. Some of the most militant practitioners of ageism can be the aged themselves. "I'm too old" is a common reply to questions about pursuing a new hobby, schooling, or work. Often these people cite expectations that they would not be able to keep up in class or to work long enough to make their efforts worthwhile. The unspoken sense is that the person is either not smart enough to compete with or would be getting in the way of younger people. The same is often true with sexuality, almost as if physical closeness and intimacy are only for the young.

What does all this have to do with adjusting to the nursing home? If the nursing home represents for the individual and family alike the realness of aging, then it may be a time when all involved grieve the loss of things that are associated with youth: strength (mental and physical), attractiveness, power, specialness, and worth. No wonder it is a tough time.

The elderly and their children are not the only ones with prejudiced views of the elderly. Caregivers of all types may have acknowledged or unacknowledged stereotypes that affect the care they provide. Some more overt and unpleasant examples include the anger often expressed by young physicians at hospital admission of an elderly person with multiple chronic medical problems, the term "gomer" (which stands for "get out of my emergency room") applied to these people, and the sudden cost consciousness when deciding to order tests or treatment, seemingly based more on a judgment of the patient's worth than the test's worth.

Psychiatry is no exception. Sigmund Freud, the unchallenged father of modern psychiatry, expressed the view that psychoanalytic treatment of anyone older than age 50 was unlikely to be of help. Another example is more recent.

A 38-year-old psychiatrist doing consultations in a nursing home was asked to evaluate an 80-year-old, single, retired schoolteacher for behavior problems involving refusal to allow application or to apply to herself an ointment needed to control a rash in her groin area. The physician noted a history of a recent marked irreversible vision loss that had left this woman much more dependent on others. He theorized that her behavior problems were a way of asserting some control in her life and attempted to get her to confirm his theory.

The woman, after patiently tolerating this inquiry, inquired of the physician if he felt that her lifelong struggle with the urge to masturbate made her life a lie. This shed a slightly different light on the problems with the groin rash. The physician was able to educate and reassure the patient and the problem resolved.

The reader will note the absolute lack of consideration that sexual issues might be of concern to an elderly single woman. The physician's stereotyped views of this group altered his approach and might have altered her care if she hadn't been so troubled and felt that she must take the risk of describing her fears.

In the book *Old Friends*, Tracy Kidder describes a new peril of aging in America.

Ideal aging—these days also known as "successful aging," often depicted in photographs of old folks wearing tennis clothes—leaves out a lot of people. It is estimated that nearly half of all the Americans who make it past sixty-five will spend some time in a nursing home. More than a million live in nursing homes now. The celebration of successful aging leaves out all of them. Ultimately, of course, it leaves out everyone.

Everyone, including friends, family members, caregivers, and the elderly themselves, is subject to prejudices and stereotypes. These views may affect how we see and handle the move to a nursing home. Although we may not like getting old, our assumptions about it may be based more on our attitudes than on reality.

Readings

Francis P: "The Autumn of My Life." In *Songs of Experience. An Anthology of Literature on Growing Old.* Edited by M Fowler and P McCutcheon. New York, Ballantine Books, 1991, p 31–32

Kidder T: *Old Friends.* New York, Houghton Mifflin Company, 1993, p 222

Chapter 4

The Needs

Before we attempt to label the specific problems of the different individuals in the nursing home—the resident, the family and friends, and the staff—it may be helpful to discuss briefly the basic emotional needs we all have. This background may assist the reader in understanding why some things become problems.

There are many different ways to look at people and understand their behavior. One way is to look at how a person is going about meeting basic emotional needs. In his book *Motivation and Personality*, Maslow summed these up well: to feel safe and secure, to feel loved and to love, to have some sense of control or power in one's life, and to have some sense of privacy. Let us elaborate just a little.

To feel safe and secure is the most basic and important emotional need. We will sacrifice most other things to achieve this feeling. It is the emotional foundation on which we build our day-to-day lives. If this sense is absent, it is difficult to work, relate comfortably to others, or play. Our sense of security is based on many things. If we felt fairly secure during our childhood, with enough to eat, a home, and parents who watched over us and loved each other, we could face the challenges of school, making and losing friendships, and uncertainties about the future more easily. If our home was a dangerous or uncertain place, the tasks of both childhood and adulthood became much more frightening and unsure.

Elements of our current lives contribute to this sense of security as well. A home that feels familiar is important. When we travel, even if we have been to wonderful places and have had a good time, most of us will note that "It is good to be home." Why? We aren't looking forward to the laundry, bills, and other chores that await us. Rather we seek the sense of belonging, familiarity, and ownership that home means. When we move, even if it is to a newer and nicer place, it feels uncertain and uncomfortable for a while. It takes time to make a place feel like home—to get used to the locations of the light switches and the sounds that are different for each home and to find your way around in the dark. We work hard to get this feeling back by unpacking familiar furniture, pictures, and mementos as quickly as possible.

We also rely on our work to provide a sense of security. Work provides financial security, a sense of competency and being needed, and a source of friendships and social contacts. Most people note considerable anxiety when changing jobs, often far beyond the uncertainty of being able to do the work. Will I fit in? Will others like me and see me as doing a good job? These concerns affect our sense of security.

Relationships we can count on also contribute to feeling safe. The experience of unconditional love, in which we feel that someone will continue to care even if we make mistakes or can no longer do the things we used to do or look the same as when the relationship began, is enormously comforting. This may be particularly true for those encountering a major health change that affects the ability to provide the mutual companionship and support that was taken for granted. Most of us need this unconditional love reconfirmed periodically. In their song "When I'm Sixty-Four," the Beatles described this need well.

> When I get older losing my hair many years from
>   now
> Will you still be sending me a valentine, birthday
>   greetings, bottle of wine?
> If I'd been out till quarter to three would you lock the
>   door?
> Will you still need me, will you still feed me, when
>   I'm 64?

The second basic emotional need is the need to feel loved and to love. Although love is a word that is so overused in this culture that we love everything from sporting events to clothes to new tires, most of us have had the privilege of being loved by a parent or grandparent, a spouse, children, and a true friend. Each of these experiences is different. None of them is ideal. Yet each confirms our sense of worth and uniqueness in ways that make the trials, disappointments, and humdrum routine of our lives tolerable.

The need to love others is also important. The act of loving another, whether it is our recognition of our feeling, verbal expression, or behavior, reassures us that we value others and have something important to give.

A single woman who entered psychotherapy with problems of chronic depression and avoidance of commitment to relationships revealed a history of emotional neglect and conditional caring from parental figures. She was mistrustful of others and guarded her money, time, and privacy fiercely. Attempts at reaching out to others repeatedly ended badly because others didn't return her attempts with the same effort and she felt used. Progress occurred when she acquired a dog, "not a purebred, but one from the pound that no one else wants." The experience of having a living thing in her home, sharing the experience of being the most important and loved being, gave her a basis to hope for this in relationships with people as well.

Love, whether it is given or received, is the essence of the most intimate and trusting relationships we have. This experience is interpersonal. God, family, friends, and even pets can be the source or recipient of love. Because it is directed outside of ourselves, it is a link that connects us to the world around us. This connectedness helps confirm who we are and that our existence has meaning. The more sources of love in our lives, the better.

A 75-year-old married woman sought help for complaints of anxiety and depression. Her symptoms did not fit a typical pattern and were not responsive to medication. Further discussion revealed a progressive sense of isolation as her husband aged and became frail and deaf, her friends died ("It seems like the only socializing I do is at the funerals of my friends"), she reflected on her childlessness, and she noted a longstanding absence of meaningful spirituality. Treatment focused on assisting her to reestablish meaningful connections with others as she moved from an apartment to a retirement community and found a volunteer cause that directed her outside of herself.

The third basic emotional need is to have some sense of

power, control, or autonomy. The sense of this may be more important than how much control one may realistically have. This need may help us understand the pursuit of money far beyond what might be required for personal comfort or security. Title or position may hold the same attraction. Both money and title offer an enhanced sense of control or power in some part of our lives. They often provide choices where others have none. An individual who wins the lottery may continue to work, but it is a choice rather than a necessity. This person has the freedom to work. The fact that the drive for wealth or position might actually control the person and diminish freedom or autonomy may be less important than the feeling of power or control that wealth or position provides.

Most of us don't win the lottery or become president of a company. We must meet this need in less dramatic ways. A special talent, skill, or knowledge may provide this sense. This is verified when others praise us or come to us for instruction or assistance. Parenting, particularly in the early years, often gives us a feeling of importance as our children struggle with tasks we have mastered, depend on us, and look to us for guidance. This position may be difficult for parents to give up as children grow and leave. The so-called empty nest syndrome may have its origins in the loss of this role and its accompanying sense of importance and control. Our ability to make everyday decisions—what to wear, when and what to eat, what to read or watch on television, when to go to bed, how to spend our money—contributes mightily to our sense of control.

The fourth basic need is to have some sense of privacy. As much as most of us need both casual and meaningful contact with others, we also need times, places, thoughts, and functions that are ours alone. The sense that our body and mind are ours and that we choose to reveal what we are comfortable with when we are ready is basic to our sense of individuality. Once we mastered toilet training and bathing, our body became more our own. Privacy in performing these functions, and doing them successfully, was initially a source of pride and later taken for granted as we became functioning members of society. Many people can remember the humiliation of a bowel or bladder accident in early childhood or one associated with illness in adulthood.

Much of the discomfort people have in the hospital comes from the expectation that others can easily set aside this privacy. Health care professionals probe our orifices, study our genitals, inquire about the frequency and quality of our bowel movements, and require us to collect samples for study. We are required to wear gowns that cover little. People enter our room without being asked at all hours of the day and night. We tolerate these violations because we are afraid of whatever caused the hospitalization and of incurring the displeasure of our caregivers, on whom we are totally dependent. We endure it because it is a limited time and we think we have enough to gain to make it worthwhile.

The need for privacy or individuality may be expressed in the types of possessions we value and keep. Most of us have quirks, habits, traits, or behaviors that we have acquired over the years that we would be embarrassed if others knew about, yet they cause no one harm. These too we may keep to ourselves. Most of us know the pleasure of a little time to ourselves at the end of a day filled with obligation and meeting others' needs at work or at home.

Privacy confirms our uniqueness and our competence. It reaffirms that we are pretty good company for ourselves and can meet many of our own needs. It serves to reassure us that we can handle the basics of everyday living.

It is probably obvious that no one gets all four of these basic emotional needs met at the same time. The pattern is that of compromise. We tend to pursue the four needs listed above in the order they are listed. A sense of safety and security must come first. Everything is compromised for this. An example is the hospital experience described above. People fairly readily surrender a sense of privacy to maintain or regain a sense of safety and security.

The compromises among needs are usually made without much conscious thought. Rather, we choose based on what seems right. The importance of the sense of having a choice cannot be overemphasized in the ongoing adjustments we make among these needs.

Reading

Maslow AH: *Motivation and Personality.* Second edition. New York, Harper & Row, 1970, pp 35–46

Chapter 5

The Resident's Challenges

If we are to better manage the transition to life in a nursing home, we must think of the problems encountered by the person coming to live in the nursing home.

One of the most common problems faced by the new resident is the lack of opportunity to participate in the decision to enter the nursing home. In the previous chapter we noted that a basic emotional need is to have a sense of power and control. In a study reported in *The Gerontologist*, Reinardy found that both objective data and residents' perceptions suggested that more than 50 percent of residents did not participate in the decision to enter the nursing home.

There are few opportunities for new residents to feel in charge of their fate at the time of nursing home entry. In an article in *Geriatric Nursing*, Chenitz notes that factors associated with better adaptation to the nursing home include the following:

- the voluntary or involuntary nature of the move, which encompasses decision-making

- the predictability of the move and degree of control elders have over events surrounding it
- the extent of environmental change as a result of the move
- the physical and mental health of elders at the time of the move
- the degree and type of preparation for the move.

Health problems bring the person to the nursing home. These can be new and catastrophic, such as a stroke, which suddenly changes the person's life from routine self-care to being highly dependent on others. Or, they can be gradual and progressive, such as Alzheimer's-type dementia or the complex changes in vision, circulation, and sensation of the diabetic.

The adjustment tasks for these medical conditions vary with the condition and the individual. Previously healthy people must suddenly contend with the fact that they are no longer able to care for themselves. They can no longer count on their body (or mind) to do what they ask of it. Although most of us have had to come to grips with the reality that we have only limited control of our relationships and our surroundings, we have learned to count on our body and our mind to do what we ask. Health changes attack our sense of wholeness and power. Both physical changes and fear (of pain, of recurrence of a stroke or heart attack, of falling) erode our sense of security. We may look different, walk or speak differently, or need obvious physical aids (a cane or walker, a magnifying glass to read, or a wheelchair) that cause us to see ourselves differently and the world around us to treat us differently.

For those with progressive conditions, the adaptation may be more gradual and the shock of being different may be less disturbing. However, there is no gradual transition to a nursing home. You are either there or you are not. The move may attack the healthy denial that we all have about changes in ourselves.

Most of us have learned to adapt to change. Why is this move so difficult? First, the changes may be within us, as in the health changes described above. Second, multiple adaptations are demanded at the same time. A stroke victim may have to cope simultaneously with an inability to speak and walk, a move to a new environment, and the loss of the companionship of a spouse. Third, the person's ability to adapt is often impaired. Studies have shown that about 80 percent of people admitted to nursing homes may have a diagnosable mental illness. German and colleagues reported in *The Gerontologist* that more than half of this was accounted for by dementia. If our ability to focus on things, remember, learn, or understand is impaired for any reason, whether it is dementia, medication effect, depression, or anxiety, we will struggle in our attempts to master this new environment.

As we label some of the multiple changes the new resident encounters, we should keep in mind that the person going through them likely has impaired mood, alertness, or memory.

Environmental changes may be the most immediately noticeable. The individual is not at home. We have discussed how home provides a sense of comfort, safety, and security. The strangeness of the setting, particularly for the memory-impaired individual, can be terrifying. Different lighting, different smells, and different and often frightening noises assail already-fragile coping skills. To be awakened at night by yelling or someone constantly calling "Help me!" would be unnerving for anyone.

Enforced routines for eating, sleeping, and bathing decrease the sense of control and individualism for the new resident. Routine is important for most of us, but nursing home routines are seldom our routines. Few things are more basic than what we eat, when we sleep, when and how we bathe, and what we wear. We have taken these things for granted for years. In our adult lives, choosing what we eat or when we go to bed may be one of the little pleasures that make life livable. Think of the resentment and sense of loss we feel when placed on a special diet. In the article "Optimizing Mental Health in the Nursing Home Setting," Stevens and Baldwin note,

> The routinization of the institution and rigid expectations of appropriate resident behavior tend to diminish the elders' capacity for self-expression and their potential for maintaining a positive and continuous sense of self.

Loss of privacy also accompanies nursing home admission. This is one of the four basic emotional needs discussed in the preceding chapter. It is not uncommon for new residents to find themselves in a double bedroom with a new roommate. Most of us can remember the difficulties in tolerating the habits and quirks of even our closest friends (or spouse!) when exposed to them in a daily living situation. These were people we chose to be with. It may not be a surprise to learn that roommate problems are frequent sources of behavioral difficulty in the nursing home setting.

> An 80-year-old woman with moderate dementia, hearing loss, and associated paranoia required emergency hospitalization after she was discovered choking her very confused roommate. "I couldn't stand her saying those things about me," she related.

We are used to performing basic bodily functions in private. Bathing and going to the bathroom by ourselves were significant achievements in childhood and very private during our adult lives. The environment (shared bathroom, a shower room down the hall) or our need for assistance with these functions may change this privacy dramatically. This loss of privacy also applies to getting dressed. Being seen undressed or needing assistance in the bathroom, often by a caregiver of the opposite sex young enough to be a grandchild or great-grandchild, can be humiliating. Physical care of all sorts, including assistance with dressing and grooming, may be experienced as an intrusion in the individual's personal space. The most common time for a resident to demonstrate aggressive behavior is when physical care is being attempted.

The lack of privacy may also affect the opportunity for physical intimacy. Our denial of elderly sexuality is based on cultural and intergenerational assumptions and taboos. Despite normal physical changes with aging, often compounded by physical limitations with illness and the elderly's own stereotypes about sexuality, many couples enjoy physical intimacy, including intercourse, throughout their life. The desire for this may not end just because of nursing home placement. Yet expression of physical affection (whether it is holding hands or sexual intercourse) is considered private by most couples. The presence of a roommate or the unlocked door through which a staff member or a fellow resident can enter at any time may put a halt to a meaningful experience.

The loss of personal possessions is another change. Our identity and history are frequently linked with our possessions. There is little personal space in the nursing home— usually half a room, most of which is filled with a hospital bed. Even if we have downsized before—moving from a house to an apartment—there is much we can't bring. Often the move is abrupt, frequently from a hospital, and the opportunity to sort through and choose what to bring is limited. Choices may have to be left to the spouse or children. They may struggle to figure out what would be most meaningful. McCracken wrote in the *Journal of Gerontological Nursing,*

> The most frequent complaint voiced to experimenters by those about to move was not leaving friends or social activities, but instead centered around the necessity to reduce the bulk of personal belongings accumulated over a lifetime to a size which could be accommodated by a one-room efficiency apartment.

There seems to be a sex difference in types of items chosen. Men tend to choose items with material value, whereas women choose photographs and other items related to relationships. Both may serve important functions. Photographs, televisions, and furniture items were the items most often moved.

There is a loss of outside activities. Our lives are enriched by a wide variety of things. Hobbies and special interests are pleasurable things that make the humdrum, routine, and necessary chores bearable. We look forward to the trip, to getting out to the garage to work on the car or woodworking project, to trying the new recipe, or to the weekly bowling league. We do these things because we enjoy them. We often are quite good at them. The anticipation of doing them gives us a positive sense of time passing. Either the nursing home environment or the conditions leading to entering the nursing home may make continuing the activity impossible. Because the elderly often have already gone through vocational change (the empty nest, retirement), outside activities may be much more meaningful than they might seem to the middle-aged adult caught up in the frantic pace of childrearing and work. The sense of loss may be great, but it may be poorly understood by those who do not share the same interest.

Changing involvement in religious life is difficult for many. Increasing age brings with it the likelihood of encountering diminished personal power (physical changes of aging, retirement) and loss of friends through death. Both of these cause us to come to grips with our mortality. Our spiritual life may become more personally meaningful as we attempt to put life in perspective. In a culture that idolizes youth, this is one area where being older probably offers a real advantage. As church attendance by young families drops off during the summer months, the older members continue to attend regularly. Is this out of boredom or fear (cramming for finals)? Probably neither. Rather, active participation in church life meets many needs for the elderly. It is a place where widows are welcomed. It provides a setting where active participation on committees, in projects, and at social functions provides a continued sense of belonging and value. The nursing home may not alter the individual's spirituality, but it may dramatically change the person's ability to participate actively. Religion in the nursing home is often a passive experience—attending chapel services and receiving visits by ministers and parishioners that feel like hospital visits.

The loss of mobility is another change for many. There are few privileges valued more by Americans than driving a car. It signifies adulthood and freedom. Losing this privilege may evoke the sense of losing one's adulthood and freedom as well. On a smaller scale, the opportunity to walk to a nearby store for a newspaper may represent the same things. This mobility may be restricted for safety reasons in the person with dementia, whose capacity and need to walk are not impaired, but whose judgment is. Physical restrictions in mobility are also losses. Viewing the world from a wheelchair

makes a person feel smaller and more childlike. Suddenly, we
are looking up at adults again.

Friendships may change. We don't choose our family, but
we choose our friends. If our friendships are based on
shared activities, the loss of our ability to participate in an
activity may also mean the loss of the companionship that
accompanied it. There may be sex differences in this as
well. Men tend to meet social needs through shared activities (for example, fishing buddies), whereas women's relationships are based more often on shared experiences and
emotions and are therefore based more on talking than activity. This doesn't mean that one sex is more loyal or caring, but it may mean that a man's friends may have a more
difficult adjustment to visiting than a woman's.

All of these changes may lead to a sense of isolation.
New residents are likely to struggle in replacing these
losses in the nursing home. We have all had the experience
of avoiding new relationships after the pain of losing an
important person in our lives. This is an understandable
method of self-protection.

Some things make the nursing home an especially difficult place to make new friends, be involved, and accept
visitors. The new resident may be humiliated by self-per-
ceptions that being here means an inability to handle self-
care. Seeing old friends in the new setting may be
uncomfortable. Most of us have a natural fear of strangers.
If we are suffering from a dementia, faces don't become familiar and we are faced with strangers (often eventually including family and friends) all the time. If our memory is
intact, we must sort out whom we like and whom we don't.
The less privacy we have, the more inclined we are to pro-
tect it.

J.R. Kaakinen noted in "Living With Silence," a study of
residents without dementia in a nursing home, that more

than 50 percent thought they had talked less since admission. The following unspoken rules about talking were identified:

> 1) do not complain; 2) do not talk with the opposite sex and if you do keep it to formalities only; 3) do not talk about loneliness or dying; and 4) do not talk too much ...
>
> ... perceived self-regulatory statements were: 1) Residents ignore those they perceive to be senile. 2) Residents talk with those who demonstrate a willingness to talk to them. 3) Residents avoid talking with hearing-impaired residents. 4) Residents don't talk with others for fear of social consequences or to avoid a social confrontation.

If all residents operate with these taboos, fears, and constraints, initiation of conversation by residents without assistance by staff or family seems unlikely to occur.

Nursing home admission is often accompanied by changes in relationships with family members. If the new resident is married, there will be adjustments to be accomplished in several areas. We have already discussed the changes in physical intimacy brought about by health and privacy limitations. However, even in less private ways the relationship may be altered. Shared activities such as visiting family and friends, dining out, meal preparation at home, and playing cards or bingo are lost.

The mutual dependency that develops over the years is often changed because the new resident may be seen as sick and the spouse becomes the caregiver. Residents miss the opportunity to feel of value to their spouse. This may be compounded by the well-meaning spouse's attempts to make things easier by not asking anything of the resident.

Unfortunately, not all marriages are made in heaven. Nor

does longevity of the relationship guarantee that the relationship is one based on mutual love and respect. Nursing home placement may make problems more obvious.

An elderly man was seen in psychiatric consultation for questions of a personality change related to a stroke. Since admission, he had been verbally demanding, demeaning, and at times threatening to female nursing staff. He constantly expected his wife to be at his side and demanded staff to call her at all hours. Separate interviews with his wife and adult children revealed that this pattern was lifelong and unchanged since the stroke. The wife, who had managed with passive submission to minimize conflict over the years, was unable to set limits on her husband's demands until she became ill with physical symptoms (stomach problems and headaches) which effectively said "no" for her.

The new resident also may experience big changes with adult children. No matter how old our children are or how competent, mature, and independent they have become, we still see them as our children. To us they seem in need of protection, advice, and assistance. Throughout their childhood we did these things as best we could, trying to provide the safe and loving environment that they needed. Even when our children are older, we may be able to provide the praise, reassurance, and support that they need from time to time.

Parent and child may experience role reversal with health problems and nursing home entry. Suddenly it is the parent who is confused, sick, dependent, and afraid. Yet it is hard to turn to our children for the things we once provided them. The new resident may experience a sense of humiliation at the physical or mental weakness and needi-

ness that has developed. This embarrassment may show itself as rejection of the child's attempt to visit or help or may
be displayed with an angry, dependent stance in which the
child is accused of not visiting or doing enough. There may
be a projection of the resident's own feelings of decreased
worth onto the child, "After all I've done for you . . . ." The
child may have the uncomfortable sense that no matter
how much he visits, it is never enough.

Behavioral problems may occur. Although this is most
frequent in residents suffering from dementing illnesses,
other factors may contribute. (Please see examples of
marital changes on pages 49 and 50.) Behavioral difficulties take several different forms. Irritability and explosive-
ness, wandering, repetitive calling out, sexually inappropriate behavior, and resistance to routine care are
commonly reported. Our response to these behaviors is
predictable. Stevens and Baldwin describe "alienation and
avoidance of them by staff, other residents, and family
members." One of the great dilemmas faced by family
members and staff alike is the need to understand these
behaviors and what they mean to the resident. Often the
resident is unable to tell us.

> Psychiatric consultation was obtained on an elderly
> man with a long-standing history of Alzheimer's-type
> dementia. He had been noted by nursing staff to be
> more restless, to be agitated when moved, to yell at
> staff members to leave him alone, and to have a di-
> minished appetite and broken sleep pattern. At times
> he reported seeing things in the room at night. He was
> unable to communicate with even "yes or no" answers
> to questions concerning pain or mood changes. His
> past history was positive for depression and alco-
> holism. The psychiatrist recommended a low dose of

antidepressant medication. Before treatment could be started, an observant nurse's aide noted strong-smelling urine, and tests confirmed a severe bladder infection. Antibiotic medicine cured the infection and stopped the agitation coming from the discomfort that accompanied it.

Sometimes it is necessary to figure out who is experiencing the distress.

An 85-year-old man with Parkinson's disease, moderate dementia, and hearing loss had previously been seen by a psychiatrist at the request of nursing staff for "yodeling" repetitively at meals. Attempts at distraction with music and earphones were unsuccessful. A subsequent consultation for food refusal and weight loss revealed a decrease in "yodeling" but expressions of worthlessness and a wish to be dead. Antidepressant medication restored appetite and abolished depressed mood. The man returned to his cheerful but irritating "yodeling."

All of these changes may contribute to a loss of the sense of self. Although it may sound like psychological jargon, this sense has both internal and external parts. Internally, there is a feeling of integrity and consistency, belief systems that serve us well, and the belief that we can nurture and care for ourselves. Externally, there is a feeling of having a place in the world that is unique, that the world is fairly consistent, and that our relationships and skills will allow us to manage what comes along. In "The Therapists' Reactions to the Elderly," Poggi and Berland note, "The old have more than accumulated many years of experience being who they are; theirs is a crisis of an identity that has been quite well-formed."

This description of some of the things facing the individual entering a nursing home is not comprehensive. It cannot describe completely what any specific person may experience. However, if we feel somewhat overwhelmed reading it, we might be feeling just a bit of what the new resident is experiencing.

Readings

Chenitz WC: "Entry into a Nursing Home as Status Passage: A Theory to Guide Nursing Practice." *Geriatric Nursing* March/April 1983, p 92

German PS, Rovner BW, Burton LC, Brant LJ, Clark R: "The Role of Mental Morbidity in the Nursing Home Experience." *The Gerontologist* 32:152–158, 1992

Kaakinen JR: "Living With Silence." *The Gerontologist* 32:258–264, 1992

McCracken A: "Emotional Impact of Possession Loss." *Journal of Gerontological Nursing* 13:14–19, 1987

Poggi RG, Berland DI: "The Therapists' Reactions to the Elderly." *The Gerontologist* 25:508–513, 1985

Reinardy JR: "Decisional Control in Moving to a Nursing Home: Postadmission Adjustment and Well-Being." *The Gerontologist* 32:96–103, 1992

Stevens GL, Baldwin BA: "Optimizing Mental Health in the Nursing Home Setting." *Journal of Psychosocial Nursing* 26:27–30, 1988

Chapter 6

The Family's Challenges

We have spent considerable time describing basic emotional needs and applying this information to thinking about the multiple life changes and losses encountered by the new resident of a nursing home. Hopefully, this will contribute to understanding why this can be such a difficult time. However, this book is not intended for the resident, but rather for the family, friends, and professional caregivers who are involved daily with this person. Much less attention has been paid to these people than to the residents themselves.

Families are complex and dynamic. Like individuals, no two families are alike. Many things contribute to this uniqueness: genetics, number and sex of the children, educational level, financial and emotional stability, personality styles of the members, and geographic location. All of these may play parts in how a family functions. Even Beaver Cleaver, growing up in the classic middle-class, white, suburban, relatively affluent, intact home environment of the 1960s television situation comedy *Leave It to Beaver,* had to contend with an older brother who was good-looking and popular. He also had to deal with a name

(Theodore) and a nickname that would have made him the butt of teasing. His traditional family setting might well have taught him that adults play specific roles: women are nurturers and caretakers of the family and men provide material stability. Luckily, we didn't have to see him deal with these issues on screen!

Because family members are interdependent (even in adulthood), a change in the status of one (death, moving away, divorce, health problems, or moving into a nursing home) often requires significant adjustments by everyone else as well. When someone moves to a nursing home, the focus is usually on that individual, rather than the family. This may cause family members to go through the coping and adapting process in isolation.

The Spouse

The spouse may experience many of the same life changes and losses as the new resident. Companionship in shared activities and shared tasks around the home and simply being comfortably at home with someone are lost. Now the spouse must get dressed, get to the nursing home, and fit in with schedules for eating, care, and therapy. This is too similar to visiting someone in the hospital. It is certainly very different from years of a private and comfortable at-home routine.

The loss of friends who are couples is a common occurrence. Many friendships are based on couples being together. When one spouse moves to a nursing home, married friends who used to talk, eat, and play together often withdraw from the friendship.

A woman in a support group offered by a retirement community noted that, since her husband (suffering from Alzheimer's disease) had moved into the nursing care area, she was seldom invited to share meals in the community's dining area with familiar couples. She noted that widows and other women with spouses in a similar situation had tended to "pick up the slack" in her social involvement within the community. Others in the group described similar experiences.

Although the origins of this behavior vary, there may be several factors that contribute. The group above (all women) suggested that much socializing from adolescence onward had been determined by men (for example, what to do on dates or socializing with couples linked by the men's work or activities). These women, an affluent and educated group, acknowledged a passive approach to social activities. They wait to be asked.

Also contributing to this change may be the discomfort of couples who remain intact. They may feel guilty about their relative good fortune, fear that their togetherness may evoke feelings of sadness in the remaining partner, or consciously or unconsciously fear the same thing happening to their own relationship.

Although we tend to ignore sexuality and territoriality in the elderly, an unattached woman may evoke anxiety and competitiveness in the woman of the intact couple. Our culture traditionally sees women as needing to be attached to men. Perhaps this is linked to women's stereotyped role as nurturer and caregiver to children and spouse, whereas men's roles have been less linked with home than with work and activities outside the home. A woman achieves success in these roles by attracting a man. There is a steadily increasing surplus of women in the older age group as men die earlier (and also tend to marry women younger than themselves). An unattached woman may therefore seem like a threat to a couple. The natural response may be withdrawal. The woman (or man) may therefore need to develop new relationships and supports as well as to deal with the loss of companionship of the spouse. There may be a loss of role and supports for the at-home care provider. The spouse of someone with a chronic illness such as Alzheimer's disease may be seen in a care-providing role. The person may have developed a well-organized support system and arrangements with family, friends, and community resources for respite care. The move of the chronically ill spouse to a nursing home may mean the loss of this support.

The healthy spouse's life may be physically affected by the change in living situation. Many couples have developed areas of expertise within the marriage that make the relationship work efficiently. Managing money, shopping and cooking, driving, and caring for the yard are all examples of responsibilities often assumed by one member of the couple. This specialization uses different skills and interests efficiently, and it offers the individual a sense of being needed and valued within the marriage.

As we become older, we also may have to support each other physically. A person with diabetes and decreased vision may need the daily assistance of the partner to check blood sugar level and prepare the right amount of insulin. If this care provider moves to a nursing home, other arrangements must be made to provide daily medical help to the spouse. The dependence between partners who have grown old together is so complex that any health or living change in one can be catastrophic to the stable but fragile living system that the couple has developed.

Marital stress or distress is a common experience in couples when one of them moves to a nursing home. As previously mentioned, long-lasting marriages are not always blissful ones. The compromises, truces, and trade-offs that have prolonged difficult relationships may be brought out into the open when one partner moves to a nursing home.

Nursing staff requested assistance in evaluating the refusal to eat of a new resident, a woman with Parkinson's disease and progressive dementia. However, when interviewed about the resident, the staff repeatedly spoke of the angry, demanding, controlling, and demeaning behavior of the husband, who at times was suspected of physically abusing his wife as well. When the staff suggested the spouse limit visits for respite, he became belligerent, threatening, and belittling to female nursing staff. The history obtained from children confirmed the long-standing pattern of this relationship.

Nursing home placement can make a difficult situation worse. In the situation above, the spouse felt less able to control his mate and his behavior became more pronounced, to both his spouse and the staff, whom he perceived as putting themselves between him and his wife.

Guilt is probably the single most common response felt by spouses. The spouse of a new resident is often overwhelmed by guilt for abandoning a mate at a time of real vulnerability and need. Marriage vows are taken seriously by most and "in sickness and in health" is not thought of as a phrase, but as a promise. Nursing home placement seems to violate this commitment.

Several things may serve to increase this guilt. First, we fear what others may think of us. Am I seen as a selfish and uncaring person who is abandoning my spouse because he or she cannot give me what I want or need? Do others see me hiring out my responsibilities because they might interfere with my freedom or because I find them merely unpleasant? Unfortunately, people not directly involved (friends, children living at a distance) may draw these conclusions because of lack of knowledge of the situation or their denial that things could be this bad.

Second, we may fear that the above conclusions are true—that we are self-serving in our support of nursing home placement. In a new catastrophic illness, such as a stroke, there may be a sense that no attempt was made to care for the person at home. Chronic conditions, such as Alzheimer's disease, offer the reassurance of lengthy (often years) home care but may leave us wondering "Was a nursing home really necessary now?"

Third, it may be difficult to share the care with others or to turn over some of the more unpleasant and physically demanding tasks and become more of a companion again. The nursing staff is unknown and has yet to prove itself trustworthy to care for a loved one.

Fourth, there may be a sense of relief with the nursing home move. This may cause us to question our commitment to our spouse. "Do I really care if I feel this much relief?"

A fifth factor contributing to guilt is the reaction of the partner entering the nursing home. The previous chapter discussed some of the multiple tasks encountered by the new resident and reactions to nursing home placement. A nondemented person may demonstrate the spectrum of grieving behaviors. These include an initial sense of shock and numbness, denial ("I'm not that bad" or "I'll be going home soon"), anger ("You put me here!" or "You never come to visit" or "They [staff] don't know how to take care of me"), and bargaining ("I won't be any trouble. I can take care of myself if you will just take me home") before coming to some new sense of equilibrium or acceptance. Often prominent in this process is anger or blame. This may be experienced as accusations of lack of love or caring, pouting when we visit, or suffering when we leave.

The reactions of the new resident with memory impairment may be even more difficult to understand or accept. The new resident may not recognize us, may react aggressively to being approached, may not seem to care if we are there or not, or conversely, may react with great anxiety and agitation to remaining in the nursing home when we leave. These reactions evoke a sense of guilt in the spouse.

As a spouse, our reactions may be similar to the reactions of the person entering the nursing home. We may deny the seriousness or potential permanence of the move, become angry and blame the nursing home staff or our spouse, withdraw from a setting that is painful to see, or attempt to control the situation by being constantly present and involving ourselves in the details of our spouse's care. Eventually, we come to recognize this move as a necessary life change. We, too, may experience a wide variety of emotions: numbness, sadness, frustration and anger, relief, and the aforementioned guilt. Although these emotions can be painful, they are normal and usually transient, lasting several weeks to months.

The Children

> ... I now mother my mother
> when I can no longer
> mother my daughter
> who is older than I
> have ever felt myself to be.

The poem above, "Like Mother, Like Daughter," by S. S. Jacobson reflects the idea that there is probably no single relationship as important and complex as that of parent and child. There is so much to be accomplished, so much invested, and such strong and mixed emotions that the relationship is likely to be filled with distortions, conflicts, and confusion. It seems amazing that it so often turns out well.

Nursing home placement frequently stresses this relationship in ways of which we may be only partly aware. Schlepp reported that "In a lifetime, the average woman will spend 17 years caring for a dependent child and 18 years caring for a dependent parent, according to a 1988 study by the House of Representatives Select Committee on Aging." This group of caregivers is now frequently referred to as "the sandwich generation." Adult children have many physical and emotional adjustments to make.

Role reversal is one of the most common experiences. We have discussed this already from the parent's standpoint. If we are lucky, there has been a gradual evolution in the way we see each other. Children often go from idealized dependency to devaluation to acceptance of the parent as an important but fallible adult. Parents often go from idealized regard through loss of control to acceptance of their child as an important but fallible adult. Both parents and children continue to seek validation and positive regard from each other. A parent's illness or disability upsets the equilibrium of the relationship.

When people become ill or incapacitated in some way, there is a tendency for those around them to see and treat them differently. Their condition evokes a caretaking response that we usually associate with the dependency of children. We may then start to regard the person as having childlike qualities. Some of the illness symptoms and behaviors seem childlike. Needing help with walking or eating, loss of bowel or bladder control, temper outbursts, and lack of comprehension of or difficulty in speech are behaviors reminiscent of early childhood.

How do our behaviors change? Often our way of speaking changes. We may find that we speak loudly and slowly (even if there is no hearing problem), choose simple words, and speak with the same inflection that we use with small children. Our sense of our parent's privacy changes. Yet, our parents have not become children. Even an individual with significant dementia can recognize a parental or condescending tone. Our parents, after all, used it on us when we were younger. Poggi and Berland wrote in *The Gerontologist*,

> Equating the older person's physical decline to the child's physical *incompetence* ignores development and greatly distorts the relationship of physical ability to age in both groups. Because the elderly lack some degree of physical competence, we should not treat them as if they lack highly sophisticated capabilities and experience.

This role reversal is uncomfortable for both parent and child. Even though we may have come to view our parents as fellow fallible adults, we may never have seen them as physically or mentally frail or incompetent. We have not often been in the position in which our parent has been dependent on us. We may resist acknowledging this by denying the seriousness of our parent's condition. Explaining away memory or behavioral problems is common. Alternatively, we may take the things said by a parent with dementia personally, seeing the parent as much more competent than is really true.

For many adults, there are unresolved issues from earlier years. Children who were victims of abuse or neglect may suddenly find themselves being called on to provide the support, protection, caring, or continued interest that they didn't receive during childhood. These individuals may find that they have difficulty doing such things in general (in the absence of appropriate modeling), and to be expected to do them for the abusive or neglecting parent may be particularly discomforting. Not only may such a person have less ability to care but the person also may find that being in a position of power evokes strong reactions.

> A middle-aged woman with long-standing anxiety and depression found herself traumatized by her mother's failing memory and nursing home placement. Her mother's unhappiness during the adjustment reevoked for the woman a long-standing sense of helplessness and anger at not being able to win her mother's approval. Her mother's lack of recognition of the woman's identity was experienced as even more proof that her mother had little regard for her. She responded by mimicking her mother's behavior—withdrawing and withholding love.

Although the woman described above was in a position of power (able to choose to withdraw), it did not bring with it satisfaction but, rather, guilt that she was doing what she had hated having done to her.

Not all of our reactions are unconscious residuals from our past. Often they spring from an inequitable distribution of responsibility among the siblings. There are usually reasons why the responsibilities of care are not or cannot be divided equally. Geography is one. Physical proximity to the parent means the individual may have more of the responsibilities for frequent visiting, speaking with nursing staff, shopping, handling finances, and communicating with other family members. These burdens are added to already busy schedules. Gender is another reason. In our society, women are traditionally seen as caregivers. There is often an unspoken expectation that the most geographically close woman will provide the care, even if this woman is the resident's daughter-in-law. Marital status also may be given as a reason for one sibling shouldering the caretaking load. A single or divorced daughter is often perceived as having fewer other responsibilities. This may be far from the truth. Schlepp noted in an article "Elder Care. Caregiving—Learning to Cope, Learning the Options," "Tension results when adult children did not freely choose to become caregivers."

The primary caregiver has a number of tasks to accomplish. First, the person must fit the time-consuming extras of caretaking into an already busy schedule. Every visit involves trips to and from the nursing home. These visits usually are not at the convenience of the visitor. The resident's schedule involves meals at specific times, therapies, rest, naps, bathing, and often early bedtimes. There are multiple time-consuming tasks that do not involve visiting. The burden of paperwork (for example, forms, taxes, finances) brings little sense of reward. Doing our own paperwork is tedious enough. Laundry, shopping for clothes and incidentals, and appointments with physicians all consume time we don't have to spare.

Communication with siblings at a distance is also a task. It is often the expectation of others that the person on site will keep others informed on the condition of their parent. In addition to the time required, the opportunity for poor communication is great. The sibling at a distance may feel that the person on site has too much control and may attempt to advise or to run things from a distance. The origins of this behavior may be multiple. Children tend to resent a special or unique relationship between a sibling and a parent. Even though this relationship may be a burdensome one in reality, it may not seem that way from a distance. The sibling at a distance may feel guilty for not providing more help and try to undo this by advising or criticizing the person on site. The sibling's opportunity to deny the seriousness of the parent's problems increases with distance. This may lead to resistance to the necessity of nursing home placement and medical decisions (including how aggressively to treat potentially terminal conditions).

The estate may be an arena in which siblings battle for control. Everyone who remembers childhood or has had children can attest to the focus on fairness throughout the life cycle. Kids compare and complain about portion sizes at the supper table, perceived inequality of time spent with or interest of parents in a sibling, or size or number of gifts at holidays. Even parents who pay careful attention to fairness tend to fall woefully short in their children's eyes. The origin of this distortion may be the fact that, uncomfortable as it may be to admit it, what we children are seeking is not fairness, but specialness. We need to be seen as unique and to stand out in our parents' eyes. Despite the maturity from life experience, the explanation to our own children that life is not fair, and the understanding that there is seldom enough time or money to meet everyone's needs, our own need to be regarded as special by our parents does not go away with adulthood.

This need is neither bad nor uncommon; rather, it is part of human nature. Biblical references abound: Cain, Joseph's brothers, and the parable of the Prodigal Son all have sibling rivalry as the source of conflict. There is an uncomfortably familiar sense of unfairness for most us in reading these messages.

Children who don't live near the parent sometimes resent the caregiver. Whether it is the perception that this person has too much influence on the parent or the fact that this person is getting to spend more time with the parent may not be important. The way we tend to measure our specialness and lovableness is by the time we spend with someone and the material gifts they provide.

The estate of the parent in the nursing home may become the final battleground on which siblings wrestle for proof of this love in a tangible (and therefore believable) way. Often the result is the same as comparing portion sizes at the supper table—everyone else's serving seems somehow larger. The conflict and resentment that can arise over this can sour sibling relationships for years.

A final task often encountered by children during a parent's move to a nursing home is confronting our own aging and mortality. Denial of the inevitability of aging and death is necessary for day-to-day function. As long as we are getting along and there is nothing to remind us of these realities, our denial remains intact. It is attacked by life events: certain birthdays, permanent health changes, moving away of children, becoming a grandparent, retirement, parents selling the family home, death of a parent or sibling, or move of a parent into a nursing home. Not all of these events may be troublesome.

However, a move to a nursing home is almost always mandated by deterioration in physical or mental ability and dependence in someone we have seen throughout our lives as competent in self-care. We may respond to this by attempting to deny the extent of the deterioration or by withdrawing, because we are unable to tolerate seeing a loved one in such a state and unconsciously see ourselves as following our parent's path.

Our reactions to the caregiver role vary. Like many other stressful and difficult situations we face, this will be unpleasant at times. It is not a role that we have looked toward with anticipation, and frequently it is not something we have chosen. We do the best we can. However, as opposed to other difficult situations, the end point of the parent in the nursing home (and therefore the end of the stressful situation) is the death of the parent. This is hard for those of us who have coped with tough times by focusing on the eventual end of the tough times. Whose suffering do we wish to be over?

The guilt we feel over such questions may lead us to work frantically in the caretaking role. This is all right if it is a time-limited experience. But if the weeks become months, symptoms of so-called burnout may occur. These consist of some combination of physical symptoms (sleep, appetite, energy, bowel disturbances), psychological symptoms (vague paranoia that your parent or the nursing home staff is trying to make your life miserable, a sense that nothing in your life is under your control, resentment of your parent, feeling trapped, guilt at not doing more, and a sense of time pressure), and behavioral symptoms (irritability, withdrawal from activities and relationships previously enjoyed). In their most severe form, these symptoms can constitute a full-blown depressive illness that may require professional care.

Frequently, these changes occur gradually and we may not notice them. When others suggest we may be struggling, we may react defensively, as if we are being told we are not doing a good enough job. Recognition that we are stressed by the special demands of a parent in a nursing home is important. Ultimately, we must care for ourselves as well.

Readings

Jacobson SS: "Like Mother, Like Daughter." In *When I Am an Old Woman I Shall Wear Purple*. Second edition. Edited by S Martz. Watsonville, CA, Papier-Mache Press, 1987, pp 20–21

Poggi RG, Berland DI: "The Therapists' Reactions to the Elderly." *The Gerontologist* 25:508–513, 1985

Schlepp S: "Elder Care. Caregiving—Learning to Cope, Learning the Options." *AORN Journal* 50:228–236, 1989

Chapter 7

The Staff's Challenges

Dr. Michael Jenike, in his introduction to a book for geriatric psychiatrists, included the following poem. It was written by a nursing home resident in Scotland and was discovered after her death.

A Crabbit Old Woman Wrote This

What do you see, nurses, what do you see?
Are you thinking when you look at me—
A crabbit old woman, not very wise,
Uncertain of health, with far-away eyes,
Who dribbles her food and makes no reply
When you say in a loud voice,
"I do wish you'd try."
Who seems not to notice the things that you do,
And forever is losing a stocking or shoe.
Who unresisting or not, lets you do as you will,
With bathing or feeding, the long day to fill.
Is that what you're thinking, is that what you see?
Then open your eyes, nurse, you're not looking at me.

I'll tell you who I am as I sit here so still,
As I rise at your bidding, as I eat at your will.
I'm a small child of ten with a father and mother,
Brothers and sisters, who love one another;
A young girl of sixteen with wings on her feet,
Dreaming that soon now a lover I'll meet;
A bride soon at twenty—my heart gives a leap,
Remembering the vows that I promised to keep;
At twenty-five now I have young of my own,
Who need me to build a secure happy home;
A woman of thirty, my young now grow fast,
Bound to each other with ties that should last;
At forty, my young sons have grown and are gone,
But my man's beside me to see I don't mourn;
At fifty once more babies play round my knee,
Again we know children, my loved one and me.
Dark days are upon me, my husband is dead,
I look at the future, I shudder with dread.
For my young are all rearing young of their own.
And I think of the years and the love that I've known.
I'm an old woman now and nature is cruel—
'Tis her jest to make old age look like a fool.
The body is crumbled, grace and vigor depart,
There now is a stone where I once had a heart.
But inside this old carcass a young girl still dwells,
And now and again my battered heart swells.
I remember the years, I remember the pain,
And I'm loving and living life over again.
I think of the years all too few—gone too fast,
And accept the stark fact that nothing can last.
So open your eyes, nurses, open and see
Not a crabbit old woman, look close—see ME.

This marvelous and lucid description of life experience is
significant for several things. First, it describes in simple

terms the rich tapestry of an individual's life. Second, it bluntly and evenhandedly describes her experience with aging. Third, her underlying spirit and need to continue to be seen as an individual are expressed in no uncertain terms. And fourth, this poem is addressed to her nurses. It is apparent that for this woman, how she is seen by those around her remains important.

We have attempted so far to describe some of the common difficulties in adapting to the nursing home for the new resident and the family members. Why include a chapter on the special tasks and challenges for the nursing home staff? After all, the treatment team is trained and paid to manage these difficult times in a professional and objective manner.

The nursing home is not an easy place to work. The role of the caregiving staff is complex and different than in other settings. Because of the length of stay of many residents, they become more than patients or residents, as do the family members who come to visit.

Consideration of the special tasks and roles of the staff is essential to promoting a sense of security and safety for the family who now is entrusting the care of a vulnerable loved one to others. Caregivers may find that this chapter helps describe things in a way that allows them to better understand and manage the difficulties present in this special work. Family members reading this may better appreciate the work of the nursing home staff.

There are many different jobs in today's nursing home. Dietitians and cooks, custodians, therapists (physical, recreational, speech, and occupational), nurses' aides, practical nurses, registered nurses, nurse practitioners or physicians' assistants, social workers, administrators, clergy, secretaries, and physicians are all involved in the daily work of the nursing home. Each of these people has special training and skills to offer. In an ideal world, this group forms a smoothly functioning team focused on the goal of providing the safest, most competent, and most compassionate physical and emotional care to the residents. As in any other work setting, this ideal is seldom achieved for long, despite mandated team meetings, quarterly reviews, and classes to upgrade skills. Why?

The health care team is made up of individuals. Each person, regardless of differences in age, sex, and training, is attempting daily to meet the basic emotional needs discussed in Chapter 4. Most of us realize that we are constantly adapting to changing personal, work, and social requirements. We may expect work to meet needs for socialization, friendship, a sense of worth, feelings of power or control, and love and validation. Although most of us work to pay the bills, we work at a specific job for the less obvious reasons mentioned above. What are some of the common problems encountered by staff members?

First, there are problems coming from the multidisciplinary team. Individuals trained in different skills tend to look at a specific resident or problem from different viewpoints. Different training often means different language to describe a problem and its origins and treatment approaches.

Psychiatric consultation was obtained on an elderly woman with dementia. The referring physician questioned the possibility of an "agitated depression" (a medical condition treated with medication). The social worker described the woman as having "disruptive behavior" (looking at the effects on the unit as a whole). The nursing staff described her as "just wild, looking for attention" (implying an underlying motive for her behavior).

The different viewpoints, language, and understanding of the problems are evident. This does not mean that any specific individual is necessarily more correct. In the example just cited, everyone was correct. The woman was suffering from a severe depression with much anxiety. Her frantic, repetitive seeking out of staff was attention seeking and extremely disruptive to the other residents.

These different viewpoints can lead to misunderstandings and conflict. We may feel that if others do not see things the same way we do, they are not valuing our opinions and we may respond angrily and defensively. Turf issues occur in any group with overlapping areas of responsibility and different training. We all need to feel that what we do is important. We also need to view ourselves as having skills and knowledge that are unique. When we feel that others are intruding in our area of expertise, we are likely to feel threatened and devalued. The natural response is anger and devaluation of the intruder. The threatened physician will challenge nurses' aides or family members who venture opinions about diagnosis or treatment by pointing to his or her medical degree, "And where did you graduate from medical school?" Nurses will devalue physician input by pointing out how little time is spent with the resident, "You don't see the physician around at night when the resident has been yelling for three hours!"

Authority issues compound communication and turf difficulties. We all like to feel that we have some control over our lives at work and at home. Supervisors often are seen as impeding the individual's opportunity to do a good job. Taking orders doesn't come naturally for most adults and is often experienced more as criticism than direction.

Bureaucratic and administrative requirements are a significant part of most nursing home staff members' lives.

State and federal regulations and documentation requirements provide important structure for safety and resident care. However, the cost of these measures is twofold. First, there is a decrease in the amount of time available to spend with the residents. Charting of symptoms and bodily functions and filling out forms are mandated by law. An eight-hour shift doesn't get longer to accommodate these increasing requirements. Because there is mandated physical care to be provided, social interaction is sacrificed. This may have both behavioral and mood consequences.

> Psychiatric consultation was obtained for an elderly woman for aggressive behavior toward staff. This resident suffered from a moderate dementia and hearing loss. Discussion with nurses and aides indicated a pattern in which the behavior often was preceded by busy staff approaching the patient rapidly (often from the side or back) and announcing the need to bathe or to prepare for bed. The staff developed a plan to (no matter how busy) approach the woman slowly from the front, get her attention, and announce loudly to her good ear the time and the task and to ask her permission to help. The behavior problems improved significantly.

In this situation, the staff, pressed for time and with the need to accomplish the task, fostered aggressive behavior from a frightened resident who did not know what was happening to her. Financial limitations do not allow nursing homes simply to hire more staff to allow for the increased time spent with mandated documentation. In the article "Optimizing Mental Health in the Nursing Home Setting," Stevens and Baldwin describe factors in the nursing home that promote increased dependency of residents on staff:

inadequate client-staff ratios, insufficient training of staff regarding the emotional needs and behavioral management of residents, overemphasis on the functional and physical (e.g., task) aspects of care, and over-protectiveness of residents by staff due to the fear of litigation.

The second cost is in staff morale. Mandated standards of care are necessary and often have had their origins in abuses. However, when we are told to do something, particularly something we already know, the common reaction is that others must see us as ignorant or untrustworthy to provide good care without supervision. We may find ourselves feeling more responsible to the regulations than to the residents. If so, it will be more difficult to see residents as individuals with unique backgrounds and needs.

Residents' behavioral difficulties may make the work setting for nursing home staff members difficult. The great majority of these difficulties occur with demented individuals. Most residents with dementia do not come to the nursing home because of forgetfulness, but rather because of behaviors associated with the memory loss. These behaviors are not likely to go away with entry into the nursing home, and often the behaviors become worse as the person tries to adapt to a strange and frightening new environment.

Wandering and intrusiveness are behaviors that are usually not treatable with medication. Physically able individuals need to move about and explore their environment. This activity may be dangerous (the person who wanders away from home or nursing home) or troublesome. Unfortunately, this exploration may intrude on the turf of other residents, who may react aggressively, or on the turf of the staff. Because the wanderer does not recognize having been in the same place just minutes before, these intrusions may be repetitive and increasingly irritating to staff. We may associate these recurrent interruptions with the irritating behavior of children, who seek out reassurance and interaction with maddening questioning or endless requests. If we see the motive of the resident's behavior as intentional, our response may be angry or punishing. Medicine or physical restraint is seldom effective or appropriate and often causes more problems (medication side effects or struggling against restraint) than benefits.

Calling out or yelling is often irritating to staff and at times disruptive to the entire unit. Often this behavior is not associated with distress and may serve as self-stimulation to the individual. There may be an odd fostering of this behavior. Both staff and residents tend to avoid obviously demented, agitated residents. This may result in a decrease in outside stimulation and a need for more personal verbalizations. Remember the case of the cheerful yodeler described in Chapter 5? His behavior was very irritating to the staff.

Paranoid thinking and accusations are common in early to middle dementia. Paranoia also can occur reactively in the presence of multiple losses and life changes; as a side effect of medications; as a manifestation of acute disruption in brain function secondary to infection; as a result of vision or hearing impairment, metabolic changes, or circulation impairment (stroke or heart attack); or as part of an underlying psychiatric illness. Accusations are frequently directed at staff (stealing is the most common) and can be embarrassing (requiring reporting to and investigation by administration). This causes the staff to react with caution. Attempts to explain to a resident that he or she is paranoid or mistaken usually produce an angry and defensive response. How would we respond if someone told us something we knew to be true was a mistake or mixed up thinking? Paranoid accusations also can be leveled at other residents, leading to angry confrontations and sometimes physical aggression. Family members may be the targets of this thinking and it can be particularly devastating, leading to anger, embarrassment, and avoidance.

Residents' incontinence is a common frustration for staff. Cleanup adds one more thing to do in a shift already crammed with work. If we attend to the incontinent resident in an irritated and frustrated manner, our attitude may communicate itself in a way that will only heighten the resident's feelings of humiliation. Family members are embarrassed by a loved one's incontinence. They may find that this is the moment to end a visit.

Refusing care, whether it is physical care or medication, is at best an irritant to busy staff. It may require a re-approach at a later time or a report to administration with the need to evaluate the safety and legality of care refusal and may be experienced as a rejection of the caregiver. The natural response to being rejected is to reject angrily in return. If not recognized, this might take the form of neglect (not offering care at a later time), assault (rough or abrupt handling or forcing physical care), or devaluation of the resident to other staff or family.

Lack of appreciation may cause us to feel demoralized. Although we know that it is not the resident's responsibility to make us happy or fulfilled in our work, most of us need to have our efforts acknowledged. We have been taught common courtesy ("What do you say?" "Thank you") since infancy. We say "thank you" dozens of times a day. Yet the resident we care for day in and day out may not utter a word. Or the resident may complain or accuse endlessly. This can wear us down despite our best attempts to understand the resident's limited capacity to interact.

Physical aggression is a particularly difficult aspect of behavior. For most of us, aggressive behavior has been punished and has been seen as wrong since childhood. We have had to learn other responses to threat or frustration to survive in society. We tend to view physical aggression as an expression of hostility and anger. Our usual response to it is to feel angry or afraid.

Often we have learned that the only time that physical aggression is justified is in response to aggressive behavior. As much as we hate to admit it, the experience of self-righteous anger is a pleasurable one for most of us. Perhaps this is because it is the only time that anger is seen as acceptable. Society uses this emotion to justify going to war (the trumped-up border incident justifying Germany's invasion of Poland in World War II), oppressing minorities ("The only good Indian is a dead Indian"), and retaliating against individuals who have broken the law (capital punishment).

As individuals, we experience this emotion when we feel wronged, humiliated, misunderstood, or attacked. The naturalness of our angry response can be seen in many movies and television shows that have a basic theme: an extremely bad person does an unjustified act of violence to an innocent person, after which the innocent person retaliates with justified or vengeful violence. We feel good as we watch this happen.

This description may be a long way of explaining why our response to physical aggression in the nursing home may be strong. The behavior seems unjustified. We feel attacked physically and misunderstood professionally. It may make us afraid. Some individuals with dementia remain physically strong. Yet we are not allowed to retaliate. Sometimes to justify our angry response, we distort the truth.

Psychiatric consultation was obtained at the request of nursing staff for an elderly man with Parkinson's disease because of aggressive behavior toward staff. He had been a resident of the unit for several years because of the physical problems of his illness. Recently, he had become physically aggressive during required care—slapping, pushing, and pinching. In discussion with the staff before seeing the resident, they predicted, "He'll be on his best behavior when you see him . . . which goes to show that he knows exactly what he's doing!"

This gentleman was indeed pleasant and cordial. However, he had developed a significant dementia. He was well behaved during this examination because it did not involve intruding into his physical space.

If this man knew what he was doing, then our anger toward him is justified and, therefore, an acceptable way to feel. Why would we choose to feel angry? Other emotions associated with such a situation, fear or helplessness for example, are more uncomfortable. Anger is directed outward. Anger's cousin, blame, also helps us feel in control of difficult situations. Once we have established that someone or something is to blame for something, it decreases our sense of helplessness.

Cognitive impairment is almost always present in the resident who behaves aggressively. Are we correct in assuming that residents who are aggressive are expressing hostility or anger? Not always. Residents often are responding to a sense of intrusion or threat. Physical (hands-on) care is the time most likely to be associated with aggression. Aggression toward other residents is likely to occur with physical encounters (another person is in the way of the wanderer) or when someone is perceived to be intruding on the person's private space (wandering into a room believed to be his or hers, only to find it occupied by someone else).

The other experience that frequently generates aggression is the loss of choice. Meddaugh wrote about this in the *Journal of Psychosocial Nursing.*

> Freedom of behavior is an important aspect of human life. People make decisions about actions they will take, and when, where, and how they will take them. Although behavior choices are sometimes constrained, people usually perceive personal freedom in choosing their behaviors.
>
> When freedoms are threatened or reduced, people become upset.

Earlier in this chapter, we discussed the stressfulness of having others decide or dictate things for us. Yet we seldom think of how few choices the nursing home resident has in a day. The very qualities that we value in adulthood, independence and self-reliance, are not what we value as caregivers. Compliance, quietness, and passivity in the resident make the caregiver's day easier. Parents can relate to the frustration of a young's child's desire "to do it myself!" It is so much easier and faster if we can just do it our way.

The resident's ease in adapting to the nursing home setting may be related to personality style. Meddaugh observed, "The subjects who had been labeled 'talkers' and 'doers' through family interviews did not fare as well in the institutional setting as those who had been more quiet and less involved in outside activities earlier in their lives."

The behavior of family members is another source of stress and frustration for staff. The relationship between staff and family is a complex and changing one. The new resident is undergoing a transition; the family is as well.

Many family members are interested, helpful, concerned, and aware of their own needs and vulnerabilities. They are of enormous assistance in helping the staff get to know the new resident, avoiding pitfalls that the family has already learned about, and validating the staff as trustworthy care providers to a frightened and often confused individual. Unfortunately, this is not always the case.

The absent family member is not always seen as a problem but may be particularly difficult to deal with. There are many reasons not to visit, and some of these were discussed in the previous chapter. Often the staff is left trying to explain to a distraught resident why loved ones haven't come. Our reactions to this vary with our sense of the legitimacy of the absence. If the resident is demented and doesn't remember visits, redirection and reassurance are provided. If the family member has other obligations or is in need of respite from a routine visiting regimen, we are happy to explain it or fill in as best we can. However, if we see the family member's absence as unjustified, we are likely to react judgmentally. We may communicate our anger at the family member to the resident. This can lead to trouble. If we confirm the resident's impressions that their family doesn't care to visit, we are indulging in the naturally occurring phenomenon, "misery loves company." We as staff may be feeling abandoned ("holding the bag," as one staff member put it). Our dismay is nothing compared to that of the resident, however. It becomes important to recognize our reactions and manage them in private rather than confirming the resident's worst fears. It is tempting to point out to the resident that we are caring and present whereas the family member is not. This tendency to enhance our own position with the resident at the expense of the family should be avoided. We must let our own actions serve to convince the resident that we can be trusted to be there.

The controlling family member can be problematic. Some individuals are by nature controlling and dominating. Recall the husband who had always dominated his wife and attempted to continue this pattern of behavior with his spouse and the female staff when his wife entered the nursing home (Chapter 5). Family members also may attempt to control the resident's care out of habit (they've been doing it at home), a sense of guilt or responsibility, or mistrust of the abilities or caring of nursing staff. This may be particularly true in the early days of settling in. As staff, we may be aware of our competence, but we have yet to prove ourselves to the family. This mistrust may be different than in the acute care hospital setting. In that setting, new or acute flares of medical conditions threaten the patient. As we have noted, most of us are willing to sacrifice a sense of control for a sense of security. However, once a medical condition has stabilized, the need to feel in control reappears. The transition to a nursing home tends to imply to family members that a condition is stable. Because the nursing home is staffed differently (fewer registered nurses and physicians), family may feel that their loved one may not receive the same level of care as in the hospital. They may become more watchful and critical.

Complaining takes various forms, but a complaint does not make a complainer. Family members' concerns need to be considered carefully. We know that there are things we can do better, things we miss or don't know, and things that are difficult over which we may have little control. However, a pattern of complaining can be frustrating and demoralizing. Cornelia Poer, a social worker with the Duke University Family Support Program, describes several types of complainers.

1. The Constant Complainer, who finds fault with everything even if it is done correctly (for example, "The pillow isn't fluffed right.")

2. The Know-It-All, who knows everything and shares this knowledge at every opportunity (for example, "Daddy wants to take a nap in the afternoon.")

3. The Backstabber, who implies that others are not doing their job and tempts you to criticize fellow staff.

4. The Dictator, who sees only one way to do it, telling you how to do your job (for example, "Daddy must have his shoes on before he eats breakfast, even if he is in bed.")

5. The Competitor, who sees the resident's care as a contest that one person can win (for example, "You didn't take Daddy to the bathroom like you should have—did you? If you had, he wouldn't have wet his pants. I spend half my time trying to keep his clothes clean and dry and things like this could be prevented if you did your job like it should be done.")

No one enjoys criticism. It attacks our need to feel competent, trusted, and valued. The theme in the above examples is that we are being accused of being incompetent, not knowledgeable, or uncaring. Our response is anger. This anger may be demonstrated in several ways. We may avoid the relative. We may become defensive and argumentative or even accusatory in return. We may avoid the resident or even blame the resident for the behavior of the family member. In number 5 above (The Competitor), it would be frighteningly easy to become frustrated with the resident's incontinence because of the accusations leveled at us. The resident doesn't know this but may sense the anger or frustration we feel. This may increase the humiliation the resident already feels because of the incontinence. The innocent resident pays the price.

Family members may ask us for things that we have trouble providing. They may indirectly seek absolution from the guilt they feel about nursing home placement. They may wish to involve us in family disputes involving the resident's care. They may seek advice in making difficult decisions concerning minimizing or withdrawing more active or aggressive care. They may ask us to fill in emotional and social gaps in their lives created by the nursing home move by hanging around and chatting during a busy shift. These poorly understood and at times indirectly presented needs are difficult to address. We may not have had specific training in the recognition of or response to such requests. We may not have time. Yet most of us respond, but we feel guilty or dissatisfied that we are somehow not offering enough.

Families and residents have mixed reactions to staff. They may idealize us, seeing us as knowing everything and being infallible (and therefore trustworthy). They may see us as judgmental of their love and caring and feel a need to please us. They may see us as intruding into their special relationship with the resident. They may see us as punitive jailers who prevent or restrict pleasurable pursuits (sweets to the diabetic, tobacco, etc.). They may see us as potentially vengeful if angered. Residents and family members may fear retaliation by staff for misbehavior, and this fear may impede the willingness to ask questions, express concerns, or ask for help. We are busy. Families may not want to bother us with their information or concerns. It is up to us to initiate and invite approach by concerned family. In an article in the *Journal of Gerontological Nursing*, Mikhail notes,

Family members often act out guilt and unresolved family conflicts in the nursing home setting. This places a terrible burden on the resident, who is already struggling with declining health and adaptation to a strange new world. Residents may feel humiliated by their offspring's behavior. They may also fear that the staff will retaliate by being abusive or omitting care.

Nursing home staff may experience a subtle sense of devaluation by the rest of the medical care establishment. Just as we may attempt to validate our worth by devaluing others within the workplace, we may find that those who work in the intense, high-tech, rapid turnover, physician-rich environment of the acute care hospital tend to look down on those who choose to work in long-term care. A frequent complaint of nursing staff at nursing homes is lack of contact with hospital staff when one of their residents is hospitalized. Despite referral forms and dismissal summaries, the lack of direct contact (even if it is over the phone) with the opportunity to question, clarify, and share information is isolating. This lack of contact implies a lack of respect of what the other has to offer. Who should initiate this contact? We frequently wait to be asked so as not to intrude or to face rejection. This is probably not a time to worry about protocol.

As professional staff, we often feel uncomfortable with the amount of emotional attachment we may experience with longer-term residents and family members. Most medical training is focused on acute care settings. We are trained to act professionally, which implies an objective and nonjudgmental attitude. There is an expectation that we will not become emotionally invested in our patients. This is bunk. We were all people long before we became caregivers. We are people before and after work. The likelihood that we can simply put aside a big part of our humanness (humaneness?) is not great, nor is it particularly desirable. It is as much our ability to empathize with the resident or family member as our training that allows us to respond in a compassionate and appropriate manner. Attention to these reactions and use of them along with training and skills will make a better caregiver.

This focus on objectivity and professional distance is particularly difficult in the long-term setting. If nearly two thirds of residents are still living in the nursing home after a year, it is beyond belief that we will not have developed a sense of investment in people we have seen so much. Residents are important to us. Like our family or close friends, we may find them irritating, delightful, humorous, and infuriating. We may also respond this way to the resident's family or close friends who visit regularly. If a resident is hospitalized, we may find ourselves worrying and calling the hospital to check on this person's condition. These attachments enrich our work. Then the resident dies.

The death of a resident may evoke the same strong and mixed emotions that family and friends feel. Yet, if we have been trained to believe that caregivers are objective and dispassionate, we may guiltily hide or attempt to suppress our reactions. There may not be the time or the opportunity to grieve or to talk with family or coworkers. There may be an unspoken expectation that death be treated clinically—call the family, call the physician, call the funeral home, fill out the papers and forms, and move on. As this process is repeated, it may start to take a toll. We may start distancing ourselves from residents and their families, and we may find work a less enjoyable place to be.

Our attitudes toward working with the elderly may affect us. We are no less likely to harbor stereotypes about being old. Usually, however, our exposure to the elderly diminishes these attitudes as we see the wide spectrum of personalities, moods, and life experiences that residents possess. We discussed some of the negative reactions to the elderly in a previous chapter. Our task as caregivers is to be aware that our biases or prejudices can affect our decision, making and our own sense that our work is worthwhile. In an article in *The Gerontologist,* Poggi and Berland describe common attitudes of psychotherapists working with the elderly that likely apply to other health care workers as well:

1. The work stirs feelings in the therapist about his or her age;

2. working with elderly people may touch upon the therapist's conflicts about relations with parents and parental figures;

3. some therapists believe that treating the elderly is useless and they cannot change;

4. some therapists may believe their skills are wasted on the elderly who are old and want to die;

5. an elderly patient could die during treatment, which would be an extreme narcissistic blow to the therapist; and

6. colleagues may not support the therapist's work with the elderly.

If we don't value ourselves or the people we care for, we are not going to be happy in our work. None of us enjoys everything we do or everyone with whom we work. However, a chronic and consistent dislike of what we do requires examination. Do we need to look at why we feel this way? Do we need to make a change for our sake and for that of those around us?

"Burnout" is a commonly used term to describe a group of symptoms that are clues that we are not doing well in our vocation. It is not a true psychiatric problem nor is it the same for everyone. Common symptoms include a sense of chronic tiredness, a sense of feeling overwhelmed (even by small things), increased irritability, a vague paranoid sense that people are trying to make life miserable, feelings of not being treated fairly, physical symptoms such as headaches and bowel problems, a dread of work, a sense of having little control over life, a feeling of being constantly behind, and a sense of isolation. In an article in the *International Journal of Nursing Studies,* Hare and associates described burnout as "an adaptation to the progressive loss of idealism, energy and purpose experienced by people working in the human services."

Not everyone experiences burnout. Some of us are more vulnerable because of our coping style. Hare and associates reported that people who tend to handle stress interpersonally, such as talking about things or seeking advice, tend to have fewer problems than those who deal with things in a solitary fashion—working harder, becoming more guarded and self-protective, and using chemicals (nicotine and alcohol). Before we can deal with symptoms of burnout, we must first recognize we are experiencing them.

It may be no surprise to those readers who have patiently read the preceding chapters involving the tasks and problems encountered by all people in the nursing home to have noted things in each section that apply to themselves. In some ways, the division in roles is somewhat artificial. All of us are struggling with change, less sense of choice and control than we need, and the need to develop a sense of safety, trust, respect, and interdependence that is necessary to get along comfortably.

Readings

Hare J, Pratt CC, Andrews D: "Predictors of Burnout in Professional and Paraprofessional Nurses Working in Hospitals and Nursing Homes." *International Journal of Nursing Studies* 25:105–115, 1988

Jenike M: *Handbook of Geriatric Psychopharmacology.* Edited by M A Jenike. Littleton, MA, PSG, 1985, pp 1–2

Meddaugh DI: "Reactance: Understanding Aggressive Behavior in Long-Term Care." *Journal of Psychosocial Nursing* 28:28–33, 1990

Mikhail ML: "Psychological Responses to Relocation to a Nursing Home." *Journal of Gerontological Nursing* 18:35–39, 1992

Poer C: " When Families Complain." In *Optimum Care of the Nursing Home Resident With Alzheimer's Disease.* "Giving a Little Extra." Edited by E L Ballard and L P Gwyther. Duke University Medical Center, 1990, pp 71–73

Poggi RG, Berland DI: "The Therapists' Reactions to the Elderly." *The Gerontologist* 25:508–513, 1985

Stevens GL, Baldwin BA: "Optimizing Mental Health in the Nursing Home Setting." *Journal of Psychosocial Nursing* 26:27–30, 1988

Chapter 8

Growth from Change

The previous chapters detailing the problems and challenges of adapting to the nursing home were not intended to depress or to overwhelm. Often we find that labeling and describing behaviors, reactions, emotions, and their probable causes make what we encounter seem less strange or unique. We may have felt that others are managing things much better than we are. It is easy to forget that when we assess how we think we are doing with how others appear to be doing, we aren't comparing the same things. Others struggling with the same emotions and concerns may see us as doing much better than they are. Because most of us are cautious about revealing our impressions or assumptions to others, we tend not to check out our reactions. We end up isolated. One goal of the lengthy description of problems and reactions is to help us recognize that we are not alone.

Another goal is to help us focus on responses. Not all problems are solvable, but the recognition and understanding of what can and cannot be done diminish the guilt we often feel. This allows us to channel our time and energy to areas where we can make a difference. Most of us have been raised to believe that if we do the right things, everything will turn out well. Unfortunately, this isn't always true. There are many examples we can recall in the decision-making process and move into a nursing home in which things haven't worked satisfactorily despite our best efforts.

Responding to a problem may be accomplished in more ways than we realize. Many of us see doing something in a narrow way. We may downplay the worth of our visits or the value of listening. We are anxious at a funeral because we don't know what to say. When we visit someone in the hospital, we feel the need to bring a gift. In these examples, it is the interest and care demonstrated by our making the effort to be with someone at a difficult time that is the meaningful gift. The art of visiting will be discussed later. The point now is that there are many opportunities and ways to assist the resident and ourselves during this time. For example, the time we are taking to learn about and better understand the problems and their causes is something we are already doing to contribute to a better transition.

Everyone does not encounter massive problems with the move to a nursing home. Many people adjust quite well. Simms and colleagues noted in a study of residents' adaptation that was published in the *Journal of Gerontological Nursing,*

> Overall, the investigators were impressed that the elderly interviewees generally were positive about their living situations. In spite of the dismal view of nursing homes portrayed by the media, this study showed that institutional living is not necessarily negative for all residents.

We have discussed the stresses of adaptation to change. However, change brings with it the opportunity for growth, better understanding, increased knowledge, a sense of mastery, and an opportunity to reexamine the things we find important in our lives. Whether we are a relative of a resident of a nursing home or a member of a nursing home staff, we may better understand what we need to do now and how we need to prepare for our own older years.

The next three chapters are divided into the opportunities and challenges for the new resident, the family member, and the staff of the nursing home.

Reading

Simms LM, Jones SJ, Yoder KK: "Adjustment of Older Persons in Nursing Homes." *Journal of Gerontological Nursing* 8:383–386, 1982

Chapter 9

The Resident's Opportunities

The new nursing home resident faces several challenges. We have discussed some of the medical, physical, mental, and emotional tasks encountered before and after entry into the nursing home. Although these can be daunting, there is no reason to believe that a person stops handling challenges and changing simply because of nursing home entry.

The new resident must continue to meet basic emotional needs (Chapter 4). The nursing home itself is designed to meet some of these needs. Residents may feel relief with the move.

> A frail, elderly diabetic woman, previously living alone, noted a marked increase in her sense of security on entering a nursing home. She no longer worried about crime in her neighborhood, whether the home health aide would be on time in foul weather to draw up her insulin, or whether her nutrition would be looked after.

Most residents seem to go through an adaptation process. Mikhail describes four phases of psychological response to nursing home entry in an article in the *Journal of Gerontological Nursing.*

1. Disorganization. During this time residents feel displaced, abandoned, and vulnerable. They may be anxious, apprehensive, or despondent, and may express death wishes.

He noted that approximately 90 percent of nursing home residents pass through this phase in 6 to 8 weeks. Those who were admitted involuntarily often struggled with continued anger and a sense of injustice.

A 70-year-old woman was admitted to a semiskilled nursing unit of a retirement community directly from the hospital where she had been treated for manic-depressive illness. Her denial of her illness was long-standing, causing noncompliance with necessary medication and multiple relapses. On follow-up interview, she idealized her place of work (which refused to have her back) and expressed much anger at the head nurse of the unit, describing her as not listening or attending to her (the resident's) needs, effectively avoiding the issues of loss and change she was facing.

2. Reorganization. This phase is characterized by attempts to find meaning in the current setting and to make it familiar and one's own. The need to find ways to give the resident a sense of control are particularly important during this time.

3. Relationship Building. The resident develops new emotional ties with other residents and staff.

4. Stabilization. The resident develops a sense of belonging in the nursing home; it effectively becomes home.

Everyone does not go through these phases in a predictable manner. Yet people do adapt. There are several factors that seem to contribute to smoother adjustment. We can assist in some phases and not in others. In an article in *Geriatric Nursing,* Chenitz describes several factors that are associated with the outcome of the transition.

- the voluntary or involuntary nature of the move, which encompasses decision-making;
- the predictability of the move and degree of control elders have over events surrounding it;
- the extent of environmental change as a result of the move;
- the physical and mental health of elders at the time of the move;
- the degree and type of preparation for the move.

A sense of choice in the decision positively influences settling in. We discussed in Chapter 4 the need to have a sense of control over our lives. The acknowledgment of the inevitability and the appropriateness of the move allows the person to be involved in the process of the move. There are things we as family members or health care providers can do to enhance this sense of choice. Some of these things are determined by the timing of the move, some by the situation, and some by the individual's condition.

The timing of the move gives us opportunities to be of help. In an ideal situation, the individual may recognize the likelihood of the need for a nursing home, research alternatives, weigh needs and preferences, and make the choice with the support and input of friends. Frequently this requires much forethought and acceptance of a situation. This may be something an aging or ill person can do for loved ones if the person is allowed to do it. Unfortunately, this may be a time when our denial of the necessity of such a decision may cause us to sabotage a relative's or a friend's attempt to maintain a sense of control and relieve us from a burden. The earlier a relative or friend addresses the potential need to make a move, the less necessary it may seem to us.

A more common situation involves the need to make a decision to pursue nursing home placement in an urgent manner. The individual has experienced a significant medical or behavioral setback. If the person is in the hospital, the time to look for or to choose a nursing home is severely limited. Options may be few and the time to evaluate them may be even more restricted. This deprives the individual (new resident or family member) of the sense of choice and may enhance the sense of helplessness that all may feel. Other common scenarios include an abrupt deterioration in behavior of an individual with dementia (incontinence, wandering, or aggression) or the death or incapacity of a caretaker in the home. Both of these all-too-common situations are busy, emotion-filled times that require multiple decisions by several people, some of whom may not be close by.

Many of us will be through the decision-making phase by the time we read this. Addressing, as early as possible, the probable need for a move to a nursing home improves the likelihood that the transition will be a smooth one. We may want to consider this in future decision-making for other relatives or for ourselves.

Validation of the rightness of the move enhances the prospective or new resident's sense of support and continued importance to family and friends. We all need the acknowledgment and approval of others, particularly at times of loss or of diminished power or control. A united front of approval by physicians, family, and concerned friends may be a great reassurance to the person facing such a big change. The physician may be able to point out the benefits for spouse and children to the prospective resident, thereby making this a giving experience.

Everyone must acknowledge that the experience may be a difficult one. If bravery is the ability to do what we should in the face of fear, then this decision and the subsequent adaptation are courageous acts for the new resident and for those who care for the person. Our desire to minimize the pain or stress of this change may do just the opposite. The new resident, going through the period of disorganization, may sense that family and friends don't want to hear about it and that expressions of sadness, frustration, or fear only drive people away.

Maintaining self-esteem requires internal and external resources. Although no one gives someone else a sense of worth or value, we all look for cues from the world around us. New residents need to experience in words and actions that they remain interesting, worthwhile, and important. The fear of being abandoned or alone is universal. It may be even more pronounced with the commonly experienced feelings of worthlessness that accompany increased dependency on others for care. In the article "Adjustment of Older Persons in Nursing Homes," Simms and associates note,

> Factors contributing to positive self-perceptions included positive feelings about past accomplishments, interactions with significant others, ability to get around, participation in meaningful tasks, helping others, and ability to do things for self.

Family, friends, and professional caregivers should see opportunity in this list.

Choosing and taking cherished possessions and mementos enhance the new resident's sense of choice, familiarity, continued sense of individuality, and historical continuity.

McCracken notes in the article "Emotional Impact of Possession Loss" that, "Items of furniture, television sets, and photographs were most frequently mentioned as the most important possessions moved." Furniture represents personal taste and comfort, television for many provides a sense of connectedness with the outside world, and photographs are reminders of our history and valued relationships. Family members often must choose the items to be moved. McCracken urges picking "possessions that support memories, that are particularly useful, and that facilitate the continuance of important roles."

Cognitive integrity enhances the chances of smooth adaptation to the nursing home setting. The opportunity to participate in discussions, choices, and explanations is more likely to occur. The ability to learn and remember makes the nursing home setting and staff familiar more quickly.

A compatible roommate can be a surprising benefit. The nursing home staff tries to make good matches, but it often takes some work. Many nursing homes are quite full, and the first available bed usually determines the initial match. The resident, family, and staff should keep trying to match individuals with similar cognitive abilities and interests as these opportunities occur. We described earlier the tendency for nursing home residents to talk less. Anna Mae Halgrim Seaver, in an essay written before her death in a nursing home and published in *Newsweek*, described the frustration of the cognitively intact resident relating to those with dementia:

> We listen to endlessly repeated stories and questions. We meet them anew daily, hourly or more often. We smile and nod gracefully each time we hear a retelling. They seldom listen to my stories, so I've stopped trying.

J. R. Kaakinen recommends in the article "Living With Silence,"

> In order to keep residents talking and assist them with adaptation, residents who talk must be placed with other residents who talk. . . . Separation of demented and nondemented residents would be useful.

Continuing to feel useful and productive enhances the resident's mood and adjustment. Most of us feel more comfortable providing help than asking for or receiving it. There are multiple opportunities for the resident to help others within the nursing home. Ingenuity and collaboration among family, staff, and resident may provide the resident with enjoyable and gratifying times. Pursuing hobbies and sharing them with others, helping other residents, and assisting family with tasks that might be done in the nursing home gives a sense of value to the person's time and efforts. Encouragement to continue to do as much moving around and self-care as possible will reap benefits despite the extra time required. The resident with dementia also may enjoy productive activities. Repetitive actions with something to show for efforts may be gratifying.

> The skilled nursing unit of a retirement community set up an "office" for a former hospital administrator with Alzheimer's disease, complete with telephone, memo pads, and "In" and "Out" boxes. This individual's agitation and wandering diminished significantly. Other residents with dementia folded towels and washcloths.

A sense of humor is an often-neglected coping and adaptation technique in the nursing home. Most of us use humor as a way of keeping things in perspective. Humor also validates that we see things in the same way as others.

We share a joke. This may be particularly important for a new resident, who may feel different from those coming to visit. Sometimes humor is an antidote to stifling routine. In the book *Old Friends,* Tracy Kidder describes a group of five residents who made the wait before mealtimes a treat.

> They used to sing only before Wednesday's lunch, when a piano player from outside would play songs on the upright. Now they began to serenade the dietary aides before almost every meal, and when the nurse's aide called out "Okay!" and the men rose and began to file in toward their table, Art would begin right on tune, "Glory, glory halle-lu-jah." Bob and Joe and sometimes Ted and sometimes even Lou would pick it up, the five men in their line, each leaning on a cane, proceeding through the dining room in slow rhythm to "The Battle Hymn of the Republic."
>
> Joe took up the rear. As the men trooped in, single file and singing, Joe suddenly felt as if he saw his companions and himself in a mirror from above, five doddering old men on canes, earnestly and carefully limping in their line toward food. Joe stopped. He leaned on his cane, threw his head back, and started laughing.
>
> "It's nice, you know," Joe said. "Art laughs, Bob laughs. Lou. Ted. I laugh. It's nice. Jesus Christ."

Family members and staff may share a humorous occurrence or marvel at the islands of wisdom in the sea of dementia of the residents.

> Emergency psychiatric consultation was obtained for a behaviorally disturbed new resident with dementia. The resident's wife was present during the interview. At the conclusion of the examination, which was lim-

ited by the resident's severe dementia, the examiner asked for the names of common objects—including a wristwatch and its dial and stem. Much to the examiner's surprise, the resident quickly and correctly named each item, although he had been unable to name his wife moments earlier. His wife laughingly explained later that the resident had repaired watches for 50 years before his retirement. Listening to her husband's unexpected answer to the examiner's question brought a brief moment of relief to a tense situation.

Opportunities for personal growth are always present. Many of us find that the increased understanding, maturity, and self-assurance that constitute personal growth don't stop at the nursing home door. Personal growth often occurs when we are faced with a challenge. Adapting to living in the nursing home certainly constitutes a stressful new time. Tracy Kidder noted of Joe in *Old Friends*,

Joe's obituary would be shorter than the prematurely written one, but his life had expanded. That was the remarkable fact. Strangely, he had changed himself in here, inside a nursing home, of all places. He'd done the opposite of what might have been predicted. One might have thought such a fiery temperament would expend itself in fury at the irritations and confinements of this place. But when his powers to act had greatly diminished, Joe had taken control of his life. He'd done so by gaining a greater control of himself. Passions still lurked in him, but they didn't rule him anymore. He still possessed his great sympathetic capacity, and through it he'd connected with many fellow residents and with almost all of the staff. He'd made himself as useful as he could. He had entered a little society founded merely on illness, and, accepting it for what it was, realizing it was all there was for him, he had joined it and improved it. He had made a lot of friends in here, and one friend for life.

As family and staff watch the resiliency, toughness, and resourcefulness of the new resident and the others living in the nursing home, it should humble us and will change us.

Readings

Chenitz WC: "Entry Into a Nursing Home as Status Passage: A Theory to Guide Nursing Practice." *Geriatric Nursing* (New York) 4:92–97, March/April, 1983

Kaakinen JR: "Living with Silence." *The Gerontologist* 32:258–264, 1992

Kidder T: *Old Friends.* New York, Houghton Mifflin Company, 1993, pp 153–154, 322–323

McCracken A: "Emotional Impact of Possession Loss." *Journal of Gerontological Nursing* 13:14–19, 1987

Mikhail ML: "Psychological Responses to Relocation to a Nursing Home." *Journal of Gerontological Nursing* 18:35–39, 1992

Seaver AMH: "My World Now. Life in a Nursing Home, from the Inside." *Newsweek* June 27, 1994, p 11

Simms LM, Jones SJ, Yoder KK: "Adjustment of Older Persons in Nursing Homes." *Journal of Gerontological Nursing* 8:383–386, 1982

Chapter 10

The Family's Opportunities

The desire of the older person to be valued . . . is expressed in the wishes of the elderly that the young share their values, want their most cherished possessions, visit them, remember them, listen to them.

—R. G. Poggi and D. I. Berland, "The Therapists' Reactions to the Elderly"

Our culture is one of action. It is a relatively young society that is used to progress, improvement, and winning. We tend to expect success, set high goals, and focus on blame (ourselves or others) when things do not go well. Are there opportunities for success and fulfillment in the nursing home setting for family members and close friends? All of us may benefit from some practical advice and some challenges to think about further.

First, we will discuss some of the practical aspects of visiting, including different types of visits and visitors and special considerations for visiting the cognitively impaired. Second, we will examine ways to develop a working relationship with nursing home staff. Third, we will describe the need and techniques for caring for yourself. Fourth, we will address opportunities for personal growth and assuming control of your own future.

The Art of Visiting

There are many things we do in our lives without formal training. We often say these things just come naturally. Examples include how to be a good parent, what to say at a funeral, or how to be a good sexual partner. Yet we often have secret fears about our ability to do these common things. These fears stay secret because we assume that we alone are ignorant; we are embarrassed to confess our uncertainty. We stumble along with good intentions, learning by trial and error.

A visit to a loved one in the nursing home may be one of these things. The person we are visiting is someone we know well. We have a shared background and experience. Yet we often feel uneasy and inept when we visit. The nursing home setting may play a part. The smells, the presence of many aged people in the public areas, and the sounds and the behavior of the cognitively impaired can be frightening. It may be hard to see a parent or spouse ill or in such a setting. We may feel that the things we say are not good enough or may make the resident feel worse.

When faced with a painful situation, our natural reaction is to withdraw. The weather, busy schedules, and concerns that visits will be upsetting to the loved one serve as reasons for us to stay away. We often have expectations about visiting—that we will be greeted cheerfully, recognized, appreciated, and invited back. This may not happen in the nursing home for several reasons. The cognitively impaired resident may not know who we are and may react suspiciously. The cognitively intact new resident may respond to a visit with resentment, blaming, sadness, or feelings of being abandoned. New medical conditions may occupy the resident's thinking. Complaints or worry about these things makes the visitor feel ineffective and unimportant.

Nothing guarantees a good visit. Sometimes we visit because of a feeling of obligation. Often visits are surprising sources of fun and strength for the visitor. There are several things to keep in mind when we visit.

First, try to visit regularly. We have all had the experience of looking forward to a special event or holiday. An expected visit allows the resident to look forward to something and thus provides pleasure far beyond the visit itself. Regular visits also provide a sense of structure and of time passing, which are familiar feelings for the resident. When we have promised a visit and cannot come, we should take the time to let the person know of the change in plans. Regular visiting has advantages for us as well. Things that become part of our routine add stability and structure to our lives. Regular visiting makes the unknown familiar and therefore less uncomfortable. In the book *Old Friends*, Tracy Kidder describes this adaptation process for Ruth, an adult daughter.

> Not many people can bear to feel their parent's nursing home is bad. But Ruth knew this was a decent place. She knew most of the staff by now, and liked them .... As for its sights and sounds, Ruth had long since grown accustomed to them, and they did not frighten her as they did some first-time and infrequent visitors.

Second, time your visit. The resident lives in the nursing home for a reason. The resident may be receiving physical therapy, have a specific schedule for eating or bathing, or be looking forward to a scheduled activity. The resident may be napping. Certain times of day or days of the week may be better for visits. The nursing home is the resident's home and we should treat it as such. Most of us would not think of stopping by someone's home unannounced at mealtime. We should check first, either with the person or the staff, to learn when would be a good time to visit. This enhances the likelihood that we will both enjoy the time together.

Third, brief visits may be better. Visiting may be fatiguing. Conversation requires concentration and attention. There is a natural reaction for the person being visited to try to be a good host or hostess. The act of coming to visit may be more important than what is talked about.

Fourth, longer visits require activities other than conversation. When we plan on being present for a longer time, we might consider alternative activities that put less emphasis on verbal and interpersonal skills. Watching television, going for a walk, doing handwork, holding hands, and giving a backrub are examples suggested by Ballard and Gwyther of companionship in which talking to each other is not the focus. For spouses, this may feel similar to times at home, where ongoing conversation was not the largest part of the relationship.

Fifth, ask the resident questions. Although the act of coming to visit is at least as important as the content of the visit, what we talk about may help communicate how we continue to feel. Interest in what the resident is doing or observing indicates that the person's life remains important. There may be a tendency to think of the nursing home as a hospital. We are likely to focus on the individual's medical conditions or problems. It is probably better to think of the nursing home as an extension of home. Current medical problems may be an ongoing source of discomfort, concern, or disability, but they are not who the person is. We should try to ask about the person and the person's observations and impressions, concerns and worries, and funny happenings. We can share our own. We should ask for opinions.

Sixth, listen to yourself. We discussed the tendency to relate to the elderly as if they were children. We should be aware of the loudness, tone, and inflection of our voice. In an article in *Newsweek*, Anna Mae Halgrim Seaver described being on the receiving end of this from staff.

Why do you think the staff insists on talking baby talk when speaking to me? I understand English. I have a degree in music and am a certified teacher. Now I hear a lot of words that end in "y." Is this how my kids felt? My hearing aid works fine. There is little need for anyone to position their face directly in front of mine and raise their voice with those "y" words. Sometimes it takes longer for a meaning to sink in; sometimes my mind wanders when I am bored. But there's no need to shout.

We might ask ourselves, "How would I feel being spoken to as I am doing?" We can find out from our loved one if we are understood by asking "Do you hear me OK?" "Do I need to speak more slowly?" "Is one ear better for you?" Often we speak loudly and use simple, childlike language when speaking more slowly would be more helpful.

Seventh, be aware of the setting. Many individuals suffer from diminished sensory capacities but are embarrassed to tell us. Conversation may be clouded by background noise in a lounge or by a television in the room. People with cataracts may find that facing a window is painful or impairs eye contact. Chairs are frequently placed in front of windows. We shouldn't be afraid to ask if we can rearrange the furniture or turn down the volume on the television.

Eighth, get to know other residents and staff. Taking the time to get to know other residents and staff by name serves several purposes. First, it makes the setting more comfortable for us. Knowing others decreases our sense of oddness and not fitting in. There will be times when, no matter how well we have timed our visit, our loved one may be unavailable (for example, toileting, taking a nap, finishing a beauty shop appointment). The opportunity to chat with staff, a roommate, or others' relatives may reassure us that the nursing home is not an isolated and lonely place. Second, the effort we extend to know our family member's new home and neighbors validates it as an important and acceptable place to be. As we become more comfortable being at the nursing home, so will our loved one.

Ninth, listening is more important than talking. Psychotherapists have been aware for years of the power of interested and nonjudgmental listening. Most of us have had the experience of having had someone we respect take the time to listen and try to understand what we are experiencing, thinking, and feeling. This experience validates our worth and the importance of what we are going through. A nursing home resident in a therapy group run by Poggi and Berland noted, "I don't know what it does, but telling your story to someone who listens makes a difference." We tend to see listening as passive (that is, not doing something). The person just quoted tells us that this isn't true.

Talking, on the other hand, may be highly overrated as helpful. It can be worthwhile to keep the resident up to date on family, friends, and previously shared activities and organizations. If we focus only on these subjects it may serve to remind the person of what has been lost. We should beware of giving advice. Most adults make up their own minds.

Tenth, try to avoid taking the new resident's complaints and unhappiness personally. The initial weeks in a nursing home will be stressful. The unhappiness, anger, insecurity, and loss felt are normal. Complaining can be helpful as long as we see it as a coping technique. It is a way of expressing and sharing pain. The most important thing to do is listen. This validates that it is a difficult time and the person is not alone.

Problems arise when we assume the burden of the person's unhappiness and try to solve it. Because it is hard to tolerate seeing someone we care about in distress, we may try to take action to make it go away. This can take the form of attempting to change things in the nursing home (roommate, schedule, medication). We may unthinkingly tell our loved ones that what they are feeling isn't true ("It isn't so bad . . ."). Then the message to the new resident is loud and clear, "I don't want to hear of your pain." We may be driven away by our own discomfort at seeing someone we care deeply about going through a tough time and our sense of helplessness to change it. The resident's expressions of sadness, sense of rejection or abandonment, or complaints of too infrequent visits can leave the visitor feeling guilty or unappreciated. In the early stages of adaptation, just listening, rather than apologizing, defending, or correcting, is likely to produce the best response.

Visiting and listening are important things to do.

Visiting the cognitively impaired has special challenges. The resident's thinking patterns, memory, and responses vary from time to time. These things also deteriorate over time. The visitor has to adjust to these short- and long-term changes. We may feel a sense of disengagement from the resident and have much guilt accompanying this feeling. If the resident no longer recognizes us, we may feel rejected. Yet continued visiting is important for both the resident and the family member.

The following guidelines for visiting the cognitively impaired may help to make our visits go more smoothly. First, don't constantly correct or reorient. Many residents with dementia have no idea that they have memory problems. Constant corrections or reminders may cause frustration and won't improve memory. If a resident does recognize the memory loss, the reminders may be painful or embarrassing.

Second, listen to irrational statements. Challenging irrational statements may make the resident withdraw or become angry. Agreeing with the statements may reinforce them. An attentive listening approach, looking for an opportunity to direct the conversation to a different subject, often works best. We must try not to be shocked by paranoid accusations. Each time someone with dementia repeats something, the person is saying it for the first time. Patience and the knowledge that the visit and conversation are important, even though the content may be repetitious, can sustain us in an otherwise frustrating experience.

Third, discuss the past. Residents with Alzheimer's disease often have a much better memory for the distant past than the present. Our inquiry into earlier times supports our interest in the person's life, and the memories recalled are usually pleasant. These times were periods of better health and more activity. Talking about these times may enhance the person's mood.

Fourth, consider taking the resident on an outing—for a drive, a meal or coffee, or shopping. Large family gatherings on holidays may be overwhelming and need to be approached with caution. Visits to the resident's former home may evoke strong reactions. Some people become agitated on returning to the nursing home. This requires going through the settling-in process again. We all feel more secure in an environment we know. The person with dementia finds this even more important. What we see as a special treat may be a frightening experience for the cognitively impaired person. It is wise to discuss excursions with nursing staff whose judgment we trust.

Fifth, consider limiting the number of people visiting at one time. Ballard and Gwyther suggested that the person with dementia may feel overwhelmed if many people visit at the same time. Often this occurs when relatives from out of town are present. These people may be more unfamiliar to the resident. The relatives are likely to be more uncomfortable with the nursing home environment and the memory decline of the resident. The things to which we have adapted and we find comfortable are new to these visitors. It is probably best for an experienced visitor to accompany the new visitors. This helps with their discomfort. It may be reassuring to the resident as well. Even if people have to take turns in visiting, it is best to avoid a roomful of talking strangers. The experienced visitor will be more aware of signs that the resident is becoming fatigued or agitated and can guide the visit accordingly.

We all would like to know if we are doing enough. Just as we fear that we won't have enough food when we entertain, our perception of how much visiting is enough is colored by worries about what others think of us. This may be particularly true in the early stages of adjustment to the nursing home. The new resident is anxious at best. At worst, he or she may be angry, confused, and overwhelmed. We look for cues from others to find out how we are doing in any new situation. If we judge the value and effectiveness of our visits by our loved one's response, we may find ourselves feeling demoralized and backing away or trying to make it right by visiting more and more. This is a time when seeking out help and reassurance from the nursing home staff may be particularly beneficial.

Working with the Nursing Home Staff

Developing new relationships with the nursing home staff may be a surprising silver lining for family members adapting to the change and loss involved in a loved one's move to a nursing home. Many of us were taught that handling things ourselves was somehow more mature and healthy. We may have been taught to keep things in the family. Our own uncertainty about how to relate to the staff may keep us at a distance from those who could provide us with education, support, and reassurance.

We discussed some of the common problems in relationships with nursing home staff in an earlier chapter. What things can we do to avoid the pitfalls of difficult reactions?

First, introduce yourself to the staff. Even this is not as easy as it sounds. We have all been taught to be cautious around strangers. Meeting new people often feels awkward. We frequently hang back and let others make the first move. Staff may feel some of this same human discomfort. Both staff and family need to put aside this natural caution for the good of the resident. If the staff recognize us and know our name and our relationship to the resident, we are likely to feel welcomed. We also are more likely to be informed by the staff on how things have gone since the last visit. We should find out the names and responsibilities of the regular staff members and inquire how to approach them with questions, concerns, and information. This will not only provide us with needed information about the structure of the unit but also demonstrate our interest in working with the staff.

Second, introduce the new resident to the staff. Staff members are skilled and knowledgeable, but they do not know the new resident as well as we do. This is particularly important if the new resident has dementia. The social worker has probably taken a thorough background history, but busy staff may not have had the opportunity to read it. Many things are helpful to staff in getting to know the new resident as an individual. Information about work, hobbies, ethnic background, level of education, and favorite interests and activities is helpful in acquainting the nursing staff with the new resident. This information may provide staff members with subjects for positive conversation during necessary care. It also may provide the staff with clues to individualize care (see the example of the former hospital administrator with dementia in the previous chapter).

Third, share with the staff things you have seen help or hinder daily care. Again, this may be most helpful for the resident suffering from dementia. The experiments we have made in finding what works and what doesn't may not have to be repeated. On the other hand, the nursing home is a different setting, and what worked at home may not work here. The key is to make an effort to talk to the staff.

Fourth, express appreciation to the staff. We all like to have our efforts acknowledged. Sometimes we fail to acknowledge the efforts of others. Most staff members work hard for limited pay. Often we save praise or appreciation until we see the results. Yet results may be hard to measure in the nursing home setting. Saying "thank you," whether for some special service or periodically just for the day-to-day efforts of the staff, can be a terrific morale booster for people doing a difficult job.

Fifth, ask for feedback from the staff. They will see things from a different perspective. Their input about visiting, including schedules, frequency, and techniques, may help us get the most from our time with our loved one. Often we feel guilty when we leave a visit or if we are absent for a while. Discussing this with staff is one way to feel reassured. When we request information from the staff, it also says that we see them as having valued expertise.

Sixth, address problems with the staff in an appropriate manner. Our loved one's care is important to us. Often we are torn between speaking up and staying quiet. We may fear how we will be seen or that our concerns will cause reprisals toward the resident. Cornelia Poer, in a 1993 syllabus entitled *The Caregiver*, provided guidelines for approaching problems in a way that is likely to get positive results.

- Ask questions and educate yourself about your concerns. Lack of understanding may make something seem to be a problem when it actually is not . . . .
- When you speak out, be clear about your concerns and identify an acceptable outcome. Generalized complaints are difficult to address because the staff does not know what it is exactly that you want. Be reasonable in what you expect and be prepared to negotiate.
- Do not wait until the straw breaks the camel's back. It is important not to let concerns build up until you reach your boiling point. Problems can usually be handled better when they are handled early by both you and the staff . . . . Do not complain about every little thing that bothers you. You may come across as someone who is hard to please, and staff may stop trying to please you if you complain too often. Try to find a happy medium.
- Talk to the appropriate staff member. Expressing concerns with one discipline about another should be avoided. Take your comments to the staff member who has the authority to address them.

- Speak with staff members whom you get along with and not those with whom you have had difficulty in the past. We all get along better with some people than with others.
- A picture is said to paint a thousand words, so be aware of your outward appearance when you talk with a staff member. If you look angry, the individual may become defensive. Take time to calm down so that what you say, and not how you look, will be taken seriously.
- Do not argue. Be aware of your tone of voice. You may look calm, but your voice may indicate otherwise. The voice can diffuse or escalate the emotional tone in the situation.
- Try not to focus on all the negatives. Make comments about the positive aspects of care. This can help create a balance. [It will also get your specific complaint/concern taken seriously.]
- Use patience and avoid excessive demands. Staff may be busy with an equally demanding task at the time. Try to put yourself in their situation to increase your understanding of their job.
- Express your appreciation to the staff when they have worked with you to resolve problems, even if you have to compromise.
- Remember, there are no winners or losers. Work together with the staff to provide the best care for your family member.

A seldom acknowledged but frequently experienced result of nursing home placement is the development of friendships between staff and relatives of residents. This occurs as we recognize that family and staff interdependence results in the best care for the resident. Mutual respect, tolerance, and affection often develop that may last for years.

A middle-aged woman related developing a relationship with the nursing staff and aides during the 3 years that her father resided in a nursing home. When he died, some staff attended the funeral. The woman noted that for some time afterward she could not return to the nursing home. When she finally did, she was greeted warmly by staff who noted, "You've been away too long." This woman then realized that she had not only been grieving her father's death but also the loss of fun and supportive relationships she had developed with the staff. Years later, although at a geographic distance, this woman and the staff still keep in touch with letters and cards.

Taking Care of Yourself

There is no way to avoid the stresses, losses, and adjustments when a family member enters a nursing home. Common experiences and responses were discussed in Chapter 5. Although some problems faced by the spouse and the children differ and will be addressed in more detail in this section, there are some common elements to keep in mind.

You must take care of yourself if you are to be counted on in the ongoing care of your family member. This is not a short-term hospitalization during which most routine things are put aside. This is not a 100-yard dash. It is more like a long walk. To cover the distance, we must pace ourselves, rest and refresh periodically, and not forget to enjoy the sights along the way.

Use of a combination of both intrapersonal and interpersonal coping techniques is the best way to manage the inevitable stresses encountered. *Intrapersonal* techniques are those within the individual. Examples include thinking things through, mastery by learning more about a situation, using relaxation techniques, setting priorities, and utilizing spirituality. Individual activities such as regular exercise, pursuit of hobbies, and maintenance of a daily routine are important in keeping physical health and a sense of balance in one's life. *Interpersonal* techniques are those involving others. They range from formal counseling to shared activities with friends. The most common techniques are talking with and doing things with others. None of these techniques work all the time. No matter how well adjusted and flexible our coping style is, it will not prevent us from encountering the normal mood responses that accompany difficult times. Recognition of what is normal and what is not is important.

The Spouse

In Chapter 6 we mentioned some of the common problems encountered by the spouse and the children during the adaptation process to a family member's nursing home placement. Let us try to address some of these now.

The loss of companionship is profound for many people. We may experience a sense of loneliness or aloneness that is hard to bear. There is no substitute for the long-standing, comfortable, and well-defined interactions of couples. No individual (now including our spouse in the nursing home) can be expected to fill the gap. We might consider several things to help deal with this loss.

Acknowledge that our reactions are real and normal. If we did not feel the loss, then how important was the relationship? In a way, the feelings of loss reassure us of the importance of the efforts and investment in a life together.

The loss of couplehood can be a big adjustment. Accept invitations from others, even when you don't feel like it. There is a natural tendency to withdraw and simplify in the face of loss or change. We may feel guilty if we go out without our spouse, particularly if we enjoy ourselves. These social experiences serve to nurture and reassure us that our company is still desired. They direct us outside of ourselves for a time.

Don't wait to be asked to do things socially. Longtime friends may be as anxious as we are about the changes that nursing home placement brings. We are raised not to be pushy or to initiate social outings, especially if we are women. Others may assume we are grieving. Take the risk and seek out continued social contact. Your friends may find this reassuring. If their discomfort continues, you will sense it.

Try to arrange your visits to your spouse to maintain the pattern of companionship before he or she entered the nursing home. Many longtime couples share time together in nonverbal ways. Going for a walk outside, watching television together, listening to music, or going for a drive are ways of being comfortably together. Some people find that doing individual things together (doing handwork or writing letters while your spouse sleeps) can feel pleasant and comfortable for both.

The loss of the role as primary caretaker is hard for some of us. This is usually more true when our spouse has had a more chronic or slowly progressive condition such as Alzheimer's disease. We may have compensated for losses in companionship by gradually settling into a different role. Because the nursing home and its staff have assumed a lot of this responsibility, we need to redefine how we spend our time or energy. The fact that we don't provide as much physical care does not mean that we care less about the family member.

Talk with the staff about the spouse. Our insights about background, personality, and quirks will be invaluable to them.

Ask the staff, "Are there specific things that I can do to enhance my family member's care?" This may help bridge the gap between home and nursing home for the resident and the family member. Is there a favorite food that would make a day special? Food and caretaking are always linked closely. Unless there are dietary restrictions, this can be an active way of being involved in the care.

This may be the time to try something new. Often we will put off things that may be important or appealing to us, particularly if a family member has required much care. We may be free to try new things that are less couple oriented. Joining a discussion group or Bible study, pursuing a neglected hobby, taking a class, finding meaningful volunteer work, getting a part-time job, or traveling to someplace you always wanted to see are opportunities that may be open. Most of them offer the chance to meet new people with common interests.

The loss of a spouse's help may require significant life adjustments. Most couples are interdependent unless a spouse has required long-standing care at home. In a setting of new or catastrophic illness (such as a stroke), there may be many new things to do or to cope with away from the nursing home. Maintaining a home, managing money, cooking, and driving are just some of the common activities that are often done by one partner in a marriage. We may feel overwhelmed when facing the need to do these things.

Ask for help when facing new tasks. We often are embarrassed to admit our lack of knowledge or ability in certain areas of our lives. We worry about bothering others with our requests. Sometimes we hope that family or friends will come to our aid without our needing to ask. Often we see family as the only acceptable source of help. Yet how often have we seen friends facing difficult times and wished we could be of help? Give your friends the opportunity to feel useful by asking them for help. Some kinds of help are going to be needed on an ongoing basis, such as yard work or driving. Other kinds of assistance may involve learning a new skill such as cooking or managing the finances. Eventually, we may master things that we thought were beyond us. We do this because we have to. We continue doing it because it helps maintain our own independence.

Look for assistance in the public sector and through volunteer organizations. We may avoid pursuing these options because of a misplaced sense of pride. Seeking help from these sources may be associated with being on welfare or taking charity. These resources are there for a reason. They are designed to help us maintain our independence.

Ask yourself, "Do I need to simplify my living situation?" Maintaining a house, yard, and one's own health may not be possible, despite seeking help as described above. The need to look toward a simpler, safer, and less-isolated living environment such as a retirement community should be considered. However, don't rush into changes in the immediate transition time of recent nursing home admission, if possible. The fewer major changes undertaken at one time the better. No one can tell any individual whether such a move is the right one to make. Some of us need to remain in our homes at all costs. Others will find that a change increases our sense of safety and gives us a sense that we are making decisions about our own future and life.

Marital stress is often high at this time. Even good relationships are stretched and challenged by so many decisions and adjustments. We have discussed the probable origins and common presentations for this in a previous chapter. Feeling irritated, abandoned, unappreciated, and isolated is common for both partners. Our spouse may not be available to work things out because of preoccupation with his or her own adjustment. This stress is uncomfortable and feels unnatural, particularly for couples who have worked well together. The natural response is to attempt to decrease the tension rapidly. This usually does not work.

Give your spouse and yourself time to reach a new equilibrium. Although there will be many common threads with the past, there will be parts of the relationship that will be different. A frantic pursuit of the old status quo in the relationship will likely lead to increasing frustration and disappointment in oneself or one's spouse. It has been estimated that a new resident of a nursing home requires a minimum of 6 to 12 weeks to adjust to the new setting. This is for an ideal case in which the resident has felt in charge of the decision, has had a choice of nursing homes, is cognitively intact, and realizes the inevitability and appropriateness of the move. These ideal cases are rare. Departures from this scenario result in longer, and at times stormier, adjustment times. Allow time to assist both of you.

Contending with guilt is one of the biggest tasks for the spouse and children of a new resident of a nursing home. Guilt is not always bad. It is a powerful motivator for many of us. There are things about this new situation that we would rather not face. Guilt may force us to do some of the things we need to do in the early stages of adjustment to a nursing home. Visiting regularly is a good example. A sense of guilt may force us to visit when we would rather deny or avoid what has happened. Later, after continued visits have helped us adjust to the new situation, we keep on visiting because it is something we want to do.

The recognition of guilty feelings and the realistic appraisal of how much is normal and when it has gotten out of hand are both difficult tasks. It may be useful to evaluate guilt by asking yourself the following questions. How much does guilt or the fear of guilt control my decision-making and behavior? How much of the time do I feel guilty? Would an objective observer perceive that I am responsible for the things about which I feel guilty? Most importantly, would my loved one want me to feel this way? The answers to these questions may provide perspective for us as we struggle with this common emotion.

Evaluation of our own emotional responses is never easy. We may need to talk through our concerns with a trusted friend, member of the clergy, counselor, or family physician.

Acknowledging and feeling our grief may well require the same internal and external responses described above. For many of us, grief is something we associate only with death. Because grief is a natural response to any significant loss, we may experience it at times we think are inappropriate. Again, recognition of our grief and its normalcy may be the most important first step in working through the feelings of loss and redeveloping a sense of equilibrium and rightness about the situation we face.

There is a particular value to group support at these times. Unfortunately, support groups are often designed for specific populations such as caregivers of those with Alzheimer's disease or those grieving the loss of a loved one by death. Many family members of someone entering a nursing home may suffer from the same powerful mixed reactions as those experiencing the changes above, yet they seem to fall between the cracks. Sometimes the social worker at the nursing home will be facilitating a group that addresses these issues. A well-run group meets several needs. By its very existence, it acknowledges that the family is going through a difficult and challenging time. Hearing others in the same boat share their mixed emotions helps us feel less alone or embarrassed about what we are experiencing. Seeing others at different stages of adaptation reassures us that this is an ongoing process rather than a way we will always feel. We may be able to help others in the group, which diminishes the commonly experienced feelings of helplessness during the settling-in process. Good groups listen, share, laugh, cry, validate, and sometimes challenge us. They don't offer a lot of advice about what we should do or how we should feel.

The Children

Nursing home placement requires many adjustments and adaptations for adult children as well. Chapter 6 described some of these. How do we go about surviving these additional challenges in a way to make this a positive experience for both our parent and ourselves?

There are many shared reactions and needs for spouses and children of the new nursing home resident. The basic principles of having a wide variety of coping techniques, maintaining a schedule, looking after one's own health, and sharing the load are pertinent. However, there are unique needs and challenges to the parent-child relationship that bear further examination.

Role reversal, caring for the person who cared for us, requires different responses than for a married couple who had an adult lifetime to develop an interdependent relationship. The cognitively intact parent has long-standing views and opinions about the children. We must remember that our parent has seen us as totally helpless, dependent, inept, and struggling to master things that our parent mastered long before. A parent may be skeptical about our dependability now. This parent needs several things from the child:

- Respect. This is communicated by acknowledging that our parent's ideas, schedules, wishes, and opinions are taken into consideration. This may take the form of finding out the time most convenient for our parent to be visited. Inquiries into our parent's views—on politics, decisions concerning care, or the celebration of special events—confirm that we continue to see the parent as having worthwhile thoughts and ideas.
- Interest. Remaining interested in our parent's observations, current and past, may be informative to us and diminishes the sense that visiting is another obligation in the busy child's life. Regular cards and letters (particularly with pictures) assure the parent of the child's continued interest.
- Dependability. When we visit on time and follow through on promises, we enhance our parent's sense of security and value.

The experience of role reversal may be more profound when the parent is cognitively impaired. Our responses may need to be more imaginative and flexible. Reisberg noted experimental evidence suggesting that the course of Alzheimer's-type dementia often mimics, in reverse order, the developmental stages of the infant (Reisberg B, personal communication). If this is the case, the standard response of treating the parent like an adult may not always produce the best result. We may find that, as the ability to understand and communicate verbally decreases, our nonverbal communication must increase. Parents can draw on their experiences. For example, we respond to frightened children with a soothing tone and by holding them.

As adults, we may feel uncomfortable initiating touch with our parents. Yet there are many ways to touch—holding hands, an arm around the shoulders, a backrub—all establish a physical contact that may be much more soothing than words that have lost their meaning.

We may have had negative reactions to seeing nursing home residents with dolls or stuffed animals. Yet these objects may provide a sense of comfort and security that can only be provided by touching a familiar object.

Unresolved issues from our own upbringing can make this a challenging time. Parents who were absent emotionally or physically, were abusive, or in other ways did not provide us with what we needed may now need us. There is no easy answer to these dilemmas. Our unresolved anger may generate a vengeful response in which we do to our parent what was done to us. In the short run, this may provide some sense of justice, but few people find this to be a satisfying conclusion to a relationship.

Letting go of the anger may be a hard task, but it's worth the effort. It involves intellectually acknowledging that things were bad, that the errors of omission and commission were usually not malicious, that blaming or repeating the past does not undo the past, and that doing a better job of caring for a parent indicates growth and change for the better. This process, for most of us, is an ongoing and incomplete one.

One of the possible consequences of this effort is increased sadness. Anger often serves as a defense against the sadness that things weren't better and that the family wasn't the happy one that others seemed to have. If these reactions are profound, then formal counseling may well be required. This should provide a safe and nurturing setting where we can explore and understand our reactions.

Distribution of responsibility among siblings is often a formidable task, as noted in Chapter 6. Recognition and acknowledgment that it is rare to have siblings equally involved in care and decision-making can assist the primary care providers and those at a distance to avoid some of the resentment and guilt that commonly are experienced.

If we are officially (power of attorney) or unofficially (geographically closest daughter) the primary care providers, the task of communicating to siblings becomes ours. It is usually worth the effort to keep other family members regularly informed.

We have become so used to using the telephone for communication that many of us have forgotten the power of the written word. Regular, chatty update letters concerning our parent's condition, activities in the nursing home, abilities, small triumphs and accomplishments, and response to letters and cards from distant siblings will make our parent's life in the nursing home seem more real. Pictures of our parent in the nursing home setting may also diminish the sense of foreignness about this new home. This approach may avoid the phenomenon of crisis communication (the hurried call announcing some new medical or behavioral setback). Regular communication lets siblings know that they continue to be important to the parent and the primary caregiver and are not involved only when something is required in an emergency.

For siblings at a distance, there are several things to contribute. Regular cards and pictures to our parent provide regular stimulation. The telephone call or letter to the sibling in the primary care role inquiring not only about our parent but also acknowledging the efforts of this sibling goes a long way to diminish the sense of isolation that each of us, in our different roles, may feel.

Time demands require ongoing evaluation and management. This is the first generation of women who have come through young adulthood with the expectation that to be fulfilled one should manage a career, marriage, children, hobbies, friendships, and one's health. Unfortunately, changes in our culture and in our spouse's behavior, although at times well meaning, have not been able to provide the support in the form of time to allow women to reasonably achieve these goals. "A 40-hour day would be nice for starters," a divorced secretary with two young children noted recently.

Acknowledge that there is not enough time to do everything. Most of us assume that if only we were more efficient, worked harder, or slept less we could accomplish everything. The recurrent reminders that we don't are then interpreted as personal failures rather than merely reality.

Set your priorities. The silver lining of this reality is that it forces us to think about what is most important. How many things do we do because we "have always done them this way"? How important are how things look and what others may think? What sort of care do my relationships (spiritual, marital, family, friends, work, and my own physical and emotional well-being) require? Different parts of our lives require different amounts of time. Because of this, there is no recipe that will work consistently. Setting our priorities is an ongoing task. Just as there is no standard way to schedule our time, there is no absolute test to let us know how we are doing. No one is entitled to feel good all the time. However, no one is doomed to feel bad all the time either. If we are getting along from day to day, with both short-term and long-term things we look forward to with anticipation, we are probably doing well enough. If we consistently suffer from the symptoms of burnout (as listed in Chapter 7) and attempts at reprioritizing are unsuccessful, then a visit with a trusted professional is indicated. The social workers in the nursing home, a member of the clergy, or a physician is a potential first source of help.

Opportunities for Growth and Assuming Control of Your Own Future

Confronting our own mortality is one of the psychological tasks that nursing home placement often brings out in the open. We discussed this as a *problem* in Chapter 6. How can this be an *opportunity?* When we acknowledge that we will age and eventually die, this usually generates much anxiety. Denial comes to our rescue, allowing us to go on about our daily lives. Yet this encounter provides us with several opportunities.

First, it allows us to evaluate what our priorities are. Where do I want to be living? What do I want to be doing? What can I do now to enhance my physical and emotional health later? What sort of relationship do I want with my spouse and children? How do I want to be remembered? These are some of the questions we ask as we think about getting older.

Second, if we examine it carefully, the fear of death is largely manifested in youth and middle age. Elderly people often make reference to death in conversation, but seldom is it with the sense of fear or tragedy that younger generations experience. Those with a significant religious faith seem at a particular advantage at this time. As we grow older, we can probably count on being less fearful as well.

Third, this encounter with nursing home placement allows us the opportunity to take control of our own aging as much as possible. As one elderly woman said, "I don't fear death, but the uncertainty of the process of dying scares me." The elderly fear immobility, incontinence, dependency, and loss of mental capacity. What have we disliked about the illness and nursing home placement process with our parent? Are there ways to spare our children some of the same difficulties? Living wills and advance directives give the family and physicians much needed guidance as to our wishes.

There are other less formal things that we can do to continue to nurture our children and care for them long after physical and even intellectual capacity has diminished. We can talk to our own children. We can share our wishes and hopes. We can tell them we trust them. We can avoid making them promise to do or not do things that no one may have control of in the future. It won't change things and leaves a potential legacy of guilt. We can tell them we want to be remembered and that their happiness has always been our hope. We can give them permission to go on with their lives. We can ask them to talk to their children.

We should expect some resistance. Just as we become uncomfortable when our parents refer to their illness or death, our children will do the same. Yet this talk may be the most caring thing we can do for our children. It also enhances our own sense of control over our destiny. By calling the shots now, we continue to be in control long after our capacity to make informed decisions is gone.

Readings

Ballard EL, Gwyther LP: *Optimum Care of the Nursing Home Resident With Alzheimer's Disease.* "Giving a Little Extra." Duke University Medical Center, 1990, p 103, 106

Kidder T: *Old Friends.* New York, Houghton Mifflin Company, 1993, p 48

Poer C: "When Problems Arise in a Nursing Home." *The Caregiver* Summer, 1993

Poggi RG, Berland DI: "The Therapists' Reactions to the Elderly." *The Gerontologist* 25:508–513, 1985

Seaver AMH: "My World Now. Life in a Nursing Home, From the Inside." *Newsweek* June 27, 1994, p 11

Chapter 11

The Staff's Opportunities

There is no easy recipe for the new resident's or family's adaptation to the nursing home. To imply that this is possible would make trivial the complex tasks and varied backgrounds of the unique individuals who come to live in this place.

Just as the residents and their families are unique, so are the individuals who make up the staff. We spent some time in Chapter 7 discussing some of the common challenges and problems encountered by members of the nursing home staff. If this setting involved only hardship and problems, few staff members would remain for long. Most staff members can remember individuals who just were not suited for this kind of work.

Are there ways to make this a gratifying and worthwhile place to work? There may be several. The nursing home provides staff with the chance to teach, help, care for others, and grow. Not every job provides these opportunities.

In this chapter we will discuss opportunities for the nursing home staff member to find satisfaction and value in a difficult job. Just as we described for the resident and family members, the need to care for oneself will be addressed.

Three goals of the nursing home staff member might include: first, to provide optimum physical care to the residents while assisting them to feel safe and secure, cared about, and important and worthwhile as individuals; second, to make family feel welcomed and included as an essential part of the caregiving team; and third, to find one's job worthwhile and interesting. Although we often fall short of such lofty goals, individual aspects of them are attainable for each of us.

Teaching

Teaching others is an enjoyable experience for most of us. To be a teacher means we have special knowledge or expertise that is of value to others. To impart this knowledge provides a sense of accomplishment.

New residents have much to learn when they come to the nursing home. Even in the best of circumstances, things can seem overwhelming. We discussed in Chapter 4 the basic need for security. In a new place this is provided by information. Familiarity takes time. We can diminish the new resident's fears by taking the time to explain things.

Names are an important part of our lives. They imply uniqueness and individuality. We need to introduce ourselves to the new resident and learn the resident's name. The resident has an even greater task: learning very quickly the names of a roommate and the many staff on whom the new resident is dependent. The single most common memory complaint of the cognitively intact elderly is remembering names of people, even those people who are well known to the individual. We have all had the embarrassing experience of blocking on a familiar person's name. If we multiply this by many new faces and considerably older age, we will have an idea of the difficulty new residents have remembering everyone's name. A friendly introduction is the beginning of a long relationship. As much as we would like to believe that we are particularly memorable, it may be more helpful to assume that the new resident will not remember our introduction and to keep introducing ourselves until we are known.

If we acknowledge to the new resident that there is an overwhelming amount of information to learn, they will be reassured that we expect to be asked the same questions more than once. This gives the new resident permission to do something the person otherwise might be embarrassed to do. Most of us feel embarrassed to ask directions or other questions. This feeling doesn't go away when someone enters the nursing home. We need to invite questions.

Nursing home policies, routines, and schedules need to be explained. The overwhelmed new resident may not retain much of this information, but explaining it serves an important purpose. We have discussed the role that routine and structure play in providing a sense of security. The knowledge that there is structure in the form of these schedules may be reassuring to the new resident, who may see the environment as chaotic and disorganized (a reflection of the person's own inner state).

Individual expectations need to be reviewed with the new resident. "Do I come to the nurse's station for medications or are they brought to me?" "Are there rules for using the telephone or for leaving the floor?" "What things should I report to the nurses?" "Who do I go to with questions or complaints?" "When should I use the call light?" Just as knowing the rules of the road or the rules of a household provides a sense of order, knowing the rules of the nursing home makes it seem less foreign and frightening.

Teaching opportunities go beyond initial orientation of the new resident to the unit. Assisting someone to increase self-care skills and independence is a gratifying experience. Many residents are coping with new physical limitations that may seem overwhelming. Although some rehabilitation work may have been done before admission to the nursing home, much of the practice, strengthening, and mastery of new ways to do common things like walk, move oneself in a wheelchair, eat, safely transfer from bed to wheelchair, dress, and use the bathroom must be done on site. The expertise and guidance of occupational and physical therapists are invaluable, but much of the practice must be done with the nursing staff.

Motivating residents is an important part of teaching. No matter what helpful information we have to impart, it will be of little benefit unless we can communicate to the resident that learning the information or skill is worth the effort.

Motivating residents requires personal interaction. It means discussion of the value of learning the task, imparting to the resident the value that it has for the resident as well as staff, and ongoing praise, validation, and support during the efforts to master the skill. It also means getting to know the person well enough to have a sense of what will be a motivation. Is a grandchild getting married? Would I like to be able to cut my own food? Would I like to be able to move easily enough that family or friends could take me to religious services? Would I like to be strong enough to take myself to the bathroom? We discover likely motivations by communicating with the resident and family.

We also need to be aware that teaching a resident skills and independence may seem like a mixed blessing to staff. The more independent the individual is, the less control the staff members have. If an individual learns to move the wheelchair without assistance, we have less control over where the person is, for example. Also, teaching takes time. Even if we are successful, it may still take the resident longer to accomplish a task such as dressing than it would if we just did it ourselves. Therefore, our incentive to teach may not be as strong as we might think initially.

Teaching family members also can be gratifying. Family can be as overwhelmed and anxious as the new resident. We discussed some of the causes and consequences of these reactions in Chapter 6. When we take the time to teach the family about the nursing home and their loved one's condition(s), it confirms to the family that we see them as continuing to be an important part of the new resident's life as well as an important part in ongoing care. This may be reassuring for the spouse or children who are struggling with guilt or loss of the caretaking role.

What types of things can we teach the family? Information about the resident's diagnoses may be extremely helpful. The likelihood is high that the family has only partial understanding or is harboring misinformation about their loved one's condition. There are several reasons for this. The pressure on busy hospital personnel may limit the time for thorough discussion of the diagnosis, prognosis, and treatment approaches. When we are anxious, we are likely to hear only part of what we are being told. Family members may be in the early stages of grieving—one of which is denial of the severity or permanence of their loved one's condition. Sometimes we can provide information in small and repeated doses that can be understood and accepted by the family. Referral back to the resident's physician for further explanation may give the family members permission to seek out more understanding.

Policies, schedules, and routines provide the family with some basic understanding of the nursing home. As with the resident, it provides reassurance that things are organized and that their loved one is being watched over. This may be particularly important for the family of the resident with dementia who has required increasingly close supervision at home before nursing home entry.

Our availability to answer questions is important to impart to the family. We are all busy in our work, and anxious family members may fear that they will intrude or upset us by asking questions. They must be given permission to do so. Just as with the resident, we need to tell the family that we know this is a time when there is too much information all at once, and that we expect that people will have to ask some questions again.

Our names and titles are important to the family. These make the staff seem less anonymous and more approachable. It also is helpful to give information about which person to seek out with concerns and that it is all right to do so. The roles of different members of the treatment team need to be explained. Otherwise, a family member with a question or concern may feel that he or she is being passed around and that team members aren't taking the concern seriously.

Explaining new medications and behaviors diminishes the family members' anxiety and makes them feel valued as part of the treatment team. This may be particularly true for new behaviors associated with the resident's adaptation to the nursing home. An explanation of the normalcy of various expressions of unhappiness, including negativism, anger, withdrawal, and paranoia, assists the family in coping with this transition without personalizing it. Sometimes the family is profoundly embarrassed by the resident's behavior or comments. It is up to us to reassure them that we are not judgmental and have seen and heard almost everything before.

Introducing the new family to other staff, residents, and families decreases the sense of isolation that is experienced in a new environment. Other residents' families are often sources of support and information. Just as we may first ask a classmate or a coworker a question before asking a teacher or a supervisor, a new family may first seek out the advice of experienced family members. By choosing the experienced family members whom we introduce to the new family, we provide them with a resource for support and information with whom we have already formed a positive working relationship.

Informing new families about activities and special events at the nursing home starts to educate them that the nursing home is much more than a hospital. Inviting family to attend and participate in the community's special and ongoing activities tells them that this is not just a place to receive medical care, but a place to continue to participate in life as much as possible.

Teaching each other is something most of us do without thinking. This usually takes the form of sharing information. Some of it is the simple report of problems, behaviors, and activities of the residents on our shift. We also may learn of family events that will affect the resident (for example, an illness that will affect visiting, a birthday, etc.). We may have discovered a technique of managing a difficult behavior that makes a resident easier to work with. Sometimes we will read an article or attend a class that provides new insights into the behavior, illnesses, or treatments that we see every day in our work. There are times when the information provided by outside experts (with the emphasis on outside) may be viewed skeptically by the floor staff. The things that we bring to our coworkers may ring more true and be more valued.

Learning

Learning in our work can be even more stimulating than teaching. Teaching implies that we already have knowledge or expertise. Learning is acquiring something new. Having more knowledge and understanding tends to provide us with a greater sense of security and power to deal with the difficult problems we face in all areas of our life, including work. We learn in many different ways and from many different sources.

Residents are probably our best teachers. By talking with, inquiring of, listening to, and watching the residents with whom we work, we learn much about their backgrounds, life experiences, fears and worries, hobbies, and pleasures. This makes the resident a person and therefore easier to care for as an individual. Remember the retired administrator with dementia who was described in Chapter 6? Her agitation diminished dramatically when the staff organized an office for her. The knowledge of this person's past work was invaluable to the staff.

Residents teach us their preferences in the routine aspects of life such as grooming, schedules, food, and bathing. They tell us or show us what they like. The more we understand these preferences and can incorporate them into the resident's daily routine, the smoother the adaptation will be for both staff and resident.

Residents also teach us about ourselves. As we watch them struggle to reestablish a sense of security, seek some sense of control over their lives, and try to find some meaning and even pleasure in life, we cannot help but realize that the gap between staff and resident is not as great as we probably originally thought. Those of us in the careproviding professions tend to use the psychological defense of intellectualization to place a safe distance between ourselves and those whose care is entrusted to us. If we identify too strongly with the residents (that is, feel as they do), we will be overwhelmed by their problems. This is one of the causes of caregiver burnout described in Chapter 7.

Yet, appreciating the individuality of the resident helps us to set priorities in our own lives. What is really important for us to do, say, work on, and enjoy while we have the physical, verbal, and intellectual capacity and freedom to devote to our goals? Despite their cognitive and physical infirmities, residents can humble us with their tenacity, their ability to experience joy in little things, and their ability to make their feelings and wishes known with great clarity.

Residents teach us to be better at our work. A learning experience with a resident is likely to stick with us much better than things we are taught at in-service lectures (or even books!), because it is associated with a real person or situation. The retired teacher with the groin rash mentioned in Chapter 3 taught me more about stereotypes of aging than many a scholarly journal article.

We learn by trying things. Most of us will be called on to make treatment decisions, often involving behavior, because some response is required. Sometimes these things work and sometimes they don't. Either way, we have learned something. Even though we may not think of it at the time, often our choice of what to do is based on previous experience.

We learn from each other. Just as we teach each other, we learn by listening and discussing problems with others who are knowledgeable.

Psychiatric consultation was obtained for an elderly woman with severe dementia for the possibility that a significant weight loss was associated with depression. There was no evidence of a medical illness causing this change. Discussion among the nursing staff at the time of the consultation revealed that the resident recently had a new tablemate for meals, a woman with marked dementia and associated yelling. The staff decided to rearrange this resident's seating. The weight loss problems resolved without further intervention.

This informal problem solving can be gratifying for the team members involved. Not only is there safety in numbers but there is also much accumulated knowledge and experience.

Learning from outside sources brings new ideas and information to us in our daily work. This experience reassures us that we are not alone in the nursing home doing a difficult job that no one else cares about. This learning can be formal (classes, in-service presentations, meetings) or informal (reading an article in a paper or magazine about Alzheimer's disease, discussion with a physician about a new medication's advantages and disadvantages). Some of the information may be new and startling. Sometimes something that we were already aware of is formalized or restated in a new way that makes it more understandable or useful. Much of what is described in this book may be in this second category.

There are a few guidelines to keep in mind in our ongoing work in the nursing home. First, a rapid change in function, alertness, or thinking is the result of an active disease process. Often, the patient with dementia is unable to tell us about new symptoms. The first clue we have to something new or different is a change in mental status or behavior. Remember the example in Chapter 5 in which a severe urinary tract infection was manifested by visual hallucinations.

Second, the resident with dementia provides some unique challenges and opportunities. We need to attempt to depersonalize the behaviors that in other settings hold significant meaning. Aggressive, irritating, accusing, negativistic, and sexually inappropriate behaviors can be thought of as clues to underlying distress or to the inner life of the demented person. If we attempt to understand these behaviors in the context of the individual's need to meet the basic emotional needs as described in Chapter 4, often with a childlike flavor, it may assist us as we contend with frustrating and at times irritating or frightening actions.

We should attempt to find (through the resident's background history and through experimentation) ways to reach, soothe, stimulate, entertain, and make secure each resident with dementia. This sounds like an overwhelming task, but it actually represents an opportunity. Because so little is expected of the resident with dementia except a steady downhill course, the small triumphs achieved—learning one's name, finding one's room, a simple helping task around the unit—can be gratifying for the resident and the staff. These things also confirm to the family that this nursing home is the right one for their loved one.

We should be aware of the behaviors associated with dementia that are unlikely to respond to medication. This knowledge makes medication therapy for behavioral problems less likely to lead to staff disappointment and the resident's detriment. Medications are neither good nor bad. Used appropriately, they can be of great assistance in relieving the distress of pain, anxiety, depression, and psychotic symptoms that are seen frequently in the nursing home setting. There is no medication that is absolutely contraindicated because of age or illness. However, both diagnosis and medication management become more difficult in this population.

Unfortunately, we often feel the need to do something when faced with difficult behaviors, particularly with our demented residents. We may turn to medication as the answer. Please refer to the cheerful yodeler in Chapter 5 as an example. Dr. Gabe Maletta has compiled a list of frustrating behaviors that usually do not respond to medication treatment as long as they are not associated with depression, anxiety, delusion, or hallucination.

- Wandering without aim; pacing.
- Inappropriate ambulation into other rooms, beds.
- Inappropriate, insulting, hostile, or obnoxious verbalizing (including incoherence, weird laughter or crying, calling out, cursing, strange noises or screaming).
- Annoying activities (touching, hugging, unreasonable requests, invading someone's personal space, banging a walker, constant repetitive tapping, rocking, etc.).
- Hypersexuality (verbal or physical).
- Inappropriate sexual activities (including public masturbation, exposing oneself).
- Willfulness, negativism, constant complaining or other difficult personality traits (including refusing treatments, medications, or cares or refusing to eat).
- Hoarding materials (pencils, straws, cups, clothes, etc.—from other patient rooms, nursing station, med carts, etc.).
- Appropriating ("stealing") items from other patients and staff (glasses, teeth, pens, etc.).
- Inappropriate urination/defecation (including smearing feces).
- Inappropriate undressing/dressing.
- Constant or repetitive comments or questions.
- Constant unwarranted requests (for help or attention).
- Prolonged repetition of words/sentences.
- Hiding things.
- Pushing a wheelchair-bound patient.
- Tearing things; flushing items down toilet.

- Putting oneself or someone else in a hazardous situation/place.
- Eating or drinking inedible objects (including feces).
- Bumping into objects; tripping over someone or something.
- Tugging at/removing restraints.
- Physical self-abuse, eg, scratching or picking at oneself, banging head, removing catheter.
- Inappropriate isolation, e.g., refusal to leave room or to socialize.
- Physically disruptive (dumping or throwing food trays; lying on floor; intentional falling).
- Etc.

This somewhat disheartening list seems to imply that nothing can be done. However, the possibility that anxiety or depression might contribute to the intensity of some of these behaviors may warrant consultation or further evaluation.

Patience is not only a virtue but it also is often a treatment technique. We have discussed previously the natural urge for both family and nursing staff to do something to remove or improve symptoms that are painful, either for the resident or for ourselves. Just as the hardest thing for psychotherapists to say is nothing, the hardest thing for caregivers to do is wait. Residents do not stop changing just because they have been admitted to the nursing home. Physical conditions can cause the resident to deteriorate over time. The most common example may be that of senile dementia of the Alzheimer type. The ongoing changes associated with this illness mean that behaviors that may be troublesome now will not be in the future. The agitated, paranoid, accusing wanderer may progress gradually to a more passive, withdrawn, seclusive, and mute state. One is not necessarily better than the other, but we can count on the fact that behaviors are likely to change, whether the patient is treated or not.

This same principle applies to the resident who gets better. Stroke victims who gradually rehabilitate themselves may require us to alter our care approach from much hands-on involvement to that of cheerleader and occasional helper. Even the demented patient may gradually adapt to the nursing home setting. German and coworkers noted in an article in *The Gerontologist* addressing the importance of social support in nursing adaptation, that

> adaptation increases as social support increases, but this relationship varies with time in the nursing home; the longer the time in the nursing home, the greater the adaptation, if social support is high. It may be that the trauma of entering a nursing home is so great that a mediating effect is not discerned at admission. As time passes and the initial trauma diminishes, the effect of social support begins to be a significant contributor to adaptation.

The repeated references to time in the previous quotation focus on the principle that time may be our ally in dealing with adaptation and uncomfortable behaviors.

Growing

Are growing and learning the same? Not necessarily. Certainly, learning new things helps us grow. But the sense of personal growth goes beyond that for most of us.

Having a sense of mastery of some new knowledge or skill means that it becomes a part of us. Just as a new tool feels awkward and foreign in our hands, applying new knowledge takes much extra thought and effort. With repeated use, the new tool becomes increasingly comfortable to use until it is almost an extension of our hands. The same is true of new knowledge repeatedly used.

A woman sought out psychotherapy for ongoing difficulties in relationships with men, noting that she tended to choose "con artists" who were not interested in her. She would terminate a relationship, only to replace it with a similar one. She initially learned about her own low self-esteem and that her expectations of men were low as well. She eventually was able to develop a more trusting relationship with her therapist and then tried her new skills in "the real world." She noted that not only did she choose different types of men but also that the relationships were better. At the conclusion of therapy, she described feeling "like I've grown up a lot."

This example is used, not to recommend psychotherapy to everyone, but to point out that this woman, using knowledge (understanding her self-concept and what had motivated her behavior) and experience (forming a relationship based on trust in therapy), began to practice and eventually master forming her relationships in a healthier manner. She experienced this change as growth and improvement within herself.

We grow by examining our own attitudes and beliefs. This book has attempted to describe many commonly held attitudes and psychological tasks with the goal of increasing our understanding. Recognizing that the residents with whom we work evoke different emotional reactions is an important step in acknowledging each resident's individuality and our own humanity. This may lead us to a different and more satisfying conclusion about what we do and why we do it.

We grow by allowing ourselves to grieve. As we discussed in Chapter 7, a misplaced perception of professionalism may lead us to believe that the death of a longtime resident should not affect us. Grieving the loss is a formal way of acknowledging the importance of the individual in our life, often over several years. This also says that this part of the individual's life was important. It means that what we do is important. Attending the funeral or memorial service, sending a card to the family, and making a joint or individual contribution to a memorial fund are all formal ways of acknowledging our grief and the resident's importance to us. We may need to reflect on the individual's life in the nursing home, how this person made us feel, funny incidents, and the nature of this death. Some of this we do alone, and some we do with friends or coworkers. Just as the sense of time passing is important for the residents, it is also important for us. Death of a long-term resident reminds us of the normalcy of this stage of life in the whole life process.

Sharing with and supporting each other are growing experiences. When we discover that we can give and receive support from other staff, family, and even the resident, we learn that we are not alone. Many of us have been taught that independence is noble and dependence on others is weakness. This implies that we should deal with our problems by ourselves. We all have needs to be both independent and dependent. Finding out that this is acceptable diminishes our sense of isolation and the need to always appear in control.

Discovering an evolving sense of who we are and what is important to us may be a surprising outgrowth of our work. Hopefully, our work is not the only important thing in our lives, but it should be one of the important things. In previous chapters, we discussed the likelihood that we look to our work to meet needs for security, belonging, competency, worth, and socialization. What we experience at work may represent a significant part of our adult identity. We may find that, as we reflect on our work, our understanding of what we do is quite different than we originally thought it would be. Hopefully, this doesn't mean that we have become tired out, overwhelmed, and cynical. Rather, we may have found that we understand differently the importance of what we do and the setting of the nursing home.

As we watch the resident and the family struggle to reach a new equilibrium it is likely to change us and our appreciation for the importance of family throughout the whole life cycle. We may find a gradual shifting of our own priorities. We may note an understanding of our own aging and its significance that is at times uncomfortable and at other times reassuring.

Helping

Helping is an important part of what we do. Most of us help at home, at work, and in various other settings. Our motives vary. Sometimes we help because we have to—it is part of our job as an employee, parent, spouse, or friend. Sometimes we help because we want to, as in a volunteer activity or cause that we feel is important to support. In the nursing home we may be mostly aware of the help we provide the residents with whom we work. However, we also provide much help for families in less obvious ways. We looked at several examples of this helping earlier in this chapter. We also help each other. This includes the obvious ways—helping another staff member with a resident lift, a transfer, a bath, or use of the toilet and covering for another staff member during breaks or meals. Less obvious help includes the other types of support we provide in the workplace—listening to someone who has had a particularly hard shift (or has worries at home), allowing others to grieve the loss of a resident with whom they have been close, or sharing a joke.

Helping confirms that we have something to offer others. Often, our original motivation for helping isn't as important as the fact we have done it. We feel good about what we have done, whether it was our job or a volunteer activity. This is more than merely diminishing our guilt or earning our paycheck. It lets us know that we are grown up. Not all helping changes things. Much of it is repetitive. We don't cure anyone when we are changing a diaper, comforting a frightened or agitated resident, or telling the family or a coworker that what they have done or are doing is appreciated. Yet most of us would be surprised at the amount of help we have given in an average day.

Taking Care of Yourself

There are many parallels between staff and family when we look at managing our lives. There are differences as well. We should review the general considerations and the final part of Chapter 10 for information that applies here.

Our happiness at work is our own responsibility. It is not the responsibility of the nursing home administration, nursing supervisors, other staff members, families, or residents. Yet often we act as if it is. Coping with difficult behaviors, frustrating policies, not enough help, and anxious family members can sometimes make our days seem like an uphill struggle. If we constantly focus on how miserable other people or situations make us, we effectively have given up control of our work lives to others.

We should learn to recognize when we are stressed. If we don't recognize our symptoms, we are unable to do anything about them. Although the things causing extra stress vary, we are likely to experience it in predictable ways. Many of us have physical symptoms (headaches, digestive problems, fatigue, or sleeping problems), whereas others may have mood or behavior changes (feeling overwhelmed, paranoid, frustrated, or irritable). Stepping back from ourselves when we notice our symptoms is the first step in managing the situation.

What are the likely causes of our increased stress? Once we realize we are experiencing increased stress, we have the opportunity to do something about it. The first thing to do is to understand what is contributing to these symptoms. When we have identified the source, we have accomplished half of the task. Knowing the source of our discomfort enhances our sense of control. The problems we are aware of are easier to deal with than the ones we aren't aware of.

Can we do something about the problem? Even the recognition that the increased stress is caused by things outside of our control can allow us not to assume the responsibility for changing it. We often expend much energy on things over which we have little control.

Talking is a helpful technique. This is often referred to as whining or complaining. Sharing our distress with others can be helpful as long as we (or the person with whom we are talking) don't assume that the sharing will somehow change the situation. The subject can be as mundane as describing the frustrations of a specific situation or as profound as sharing the loss and grief at the death of a long-time resident.

Taking a break is important. Most of us have plenty to do. Often we choose to work through our breaks or meals because of the volume of work that is required. Breaks are in place for a reason. They allow us to not be "on" for a few minutes. We have only ourselves to care for. These few minutes can rejuvenate us beyond the actual rest they provide. They remind us that there is more to us than our work and that we as individuals are important and require a rest.

For many of us, taking a break doesn't come naturally. We often have a powerful sense that we are not only needed but are also indispensable. This may be part of the reason we chose to become care providers. However, the recognition that the unit or the residents can get along without us for a brief time is reassuring in the long run. Just as we reassure dedicated and concerned family members that their loved one is being safely and competently cared for when they are away from the nursing home, we too need to put our sense of responsibility in perspective to be of help in the long run.

The reason for emphasizing this point is that what we originally choose to do we may come to feel obligated to do. Just as the sense of choice is so important to the resident's adaptation, it is important to our own sense of autonomy in the workplace. If we feel we can't take a break, we begin to feel trapped and then resentful. It is not the residents' fault if we cannot set limits on our own sense of indispensability and obligation.

We should foster various coping styles. Just as we discussed the benefits for family of having various ways to manage the hard times, we too should cultivate solitary and social techniques. Hobbies, social activities, recreation (both individual and social), exercise, and attention to spiritual life all contribute to a sense of being a well-rounded person. People who take the time to do this are less vulnerable to feeling overwhelmed by a stress, conflict, loss, or change in any one area. Individuals who have most of their eggs in one basket experience more distress if the bottom drops out of that basket. Those of us who look to our work to provide our recreation, social life, and all of our self-worth are in a vulnerable position if something (for example, injury, illness, or layoff) keeps us from working. We might ask ourselves, "Am I expecting my work to provide more for me than I should?"

We should learn to recognize and label our emotions. The physical efforts of our work can be tiring. Feeling exhausted, overwhelmed, or burned out is much more likely to come from powerful and at times mixed emotions we experience. Managing (and particularly suppressing) strong emotions takes a lot of energy. If we can put a name on what we are feeling, we may be able to better go about choosing how to handle our reactions.

We must learn to accept our own humanity as well as that of those around us. If we cannot accept this humanness in ourselves and others, the nursing home becomes an inhuman place to work. We will feel isolated, defensive, and angry and blame others a lot of the time. Acknowledging our fallibility and limitations is not necessarily demoralizing or humiliating. When we do, we are in a position to ask for help or forgiveness for an error. We also are able to accept the fallibility of others, whether they are residents, family members, or staff members.

This acceptance goes a long way toward making the nursing home a caring and supportive place to be.

Readings

German PS, Rovner BW, Burton LC, Brant LJ, Clark R: "The Role of Mental Morbidity in the Nursing Home Experience." *The Gerontologist* 32:152–158, 1992

Maletta GJ, read at the Geriatric Research, Education and Clinical Center meeting, Minneapolis, Minnesota, September, 1991

Conclusion

This book has attempted to focus on the people of the nursing home: the residents, the family members, and the staff. Although the facility itself can be a help or a hindrance to initial adjustment and ongoing living, the people are what make it a home. We have tried to learn more about the humanity of everyone who comes here: to live, to visit, to work. Those readers who have read the entire book will probably note that there are many more similarities than differences in the needs, reactions, and tasks described for the people of the nursing home. We may find it frightening that there are so many similarities. It also should be reassuring that the nursing home setting is a place where we continue to live. All of us continue to work to meet the basic human needs that do not change. In acknowledging the humanness of ourselves (whether family, friend, or staff) and the resident, we can make this setting a more humane place to be, to work, and to grow.

Permissions

Index

A

adaptation process to nursing home
    disorganization, 98
    factors contributing to, 99–100
    relationship building, 98
    reorganization, 98
    sense of choice in decision, 99
    stabilization, 98
    timing of move, 99–100
ageism, 28–29
    elderly ageism against self, 29–30
    medical caregivers and, 30–31
    secular nature of our culture and, 29
    youthfulness of our society and, 28–29
aggression of residents, 79–82
    cognitive impairment and, 81
    loss of choice and, 82
    physical (hands-on) care associated with, 81–82
aging
    change in attitude toward, 25–26
    children's attitude toward, 25

D

L

M

N

S

U

V